Disclaimer

The publisher of this book is by no way associated with the National Institute of Standards and Technology (NIST). The NIST did not publish this book. It was published by 50 page publications under the public domain license.

50 Page Publications.

Book Title: A Bibliography of Ambulance Patient Compartments and Related Issues

Book Author: Mehdi Dadfarnia; Yung-Tsun T. Lee; Deogratias Kibira

Book Abstract: Safety in the patient compartment of ambulances is an issue of growing concern for emergency medical technicians (EMTs), paramedics, patients, and others affected by ambulances. A lot of research has been conducted by different players and much of it is scattered. As a quick reference, this report is to enhance the ability of researchers of this field to sift through a collection of standards and documents from books, journals, websites, and reports. This annotated bibliography is categorized into different fields for further ease of use. A brief abstract follows every bibliographical reference.

Citation: NIST Interagency/Internal Report (NISTIR) - 7835

Keyword: Ambulance; Ambulance Standards; Crash; Design Layout; Patient Compartment; Safety Hazards; Task Frequency

NISTIR 7835

A Bibliography of Ambulance Patient Compartments and Related Issues

Mehdi Dadfarnia
Y. Tina Lee
Deogratias Kibira

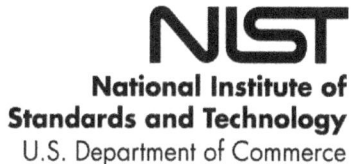

National Institute of
Standards and Technology
U.S. Department of Commerce

NISTIR 7835

A Bibliography of Ambulance Patient Compartments and Related Issues

Mehdi Dadfarnia
Y. Tina Lee
Deogratis Kibira
Systems Integration Division
Engineering Laboratory

February 2012

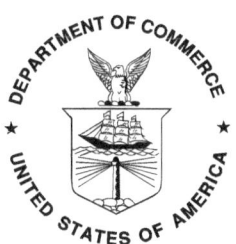

U.S. Department of Commerce
John E. Bryson, Secretary

National Institute of Standards and Technology
Patrick D. Gallagher, Under Secretary of Commerce for Standards and Technology and Director

A Bibliography of Ambulance Patient Compartments and Related Issues

Mehdi Dadfarnia
Y. Tina Lee
Deogratias Kibira
Manufacturing Simulation and Modeling Group
Manufacturing Systems Integration Division
Engineering Laboratory
National Institute of Standards and Technology
Gaithersburg, MD 20899-8260

Abstract

Safety in the patient compartment of ambulances is an issue of growing concern for emergency medical technicians (EMTs), paramedics, patients, and others affected by ambulances. A lot of research has been conducted by different players and much of it is scattered. As a quick reference, this report is to enhance the ability of researchers of this field to sift through a collection of standards and documents from books, journals, websites, and reports. This annotated bibliography is categorized into different fields for further ease of use. A brief abstract follows every bibliographical reference.

Keywords

Ambulance; Ambulance Standards; Crash; Design Layout; Patient Compartment; Safety Hazards; Task Frequency.

Table of Contents

Abstract 1
Keywords 1
1. INTRODUCTION 3
2. OVERVIEW OF THE REPORT 3
3. BIBLIOGRAPHY 5
   3.1   **Ambulance Problems Awareness** 5
   3.2   **Injury & Accident Reports** 9
   3.3   **Layout & Space Design** 16
   3.4   **Crash Test Procedures** 20
   3.5   **Other Research & Proposed Solutions** 23
   3.6   **Overall Design Evaluations and Examples** 30
   3.7   **Securing People & Equipment** 35
   3.8   **Standards & Guidelines** 42
4. ACRONYMS 47
Acknowledgements 48
Disclaimer 48

1. INTRODUCTION

Emergency medical services (EMS) personnel today face many safety issues in their working environment, the ambulance. This is because comprehensive standards for ambulance interior design, based on scientific methods, are lacking in the United States. The result is that EMS personnel are exposed to blood-borne pathogens from needle sticks, injuries from lifting and moving patients, attacks by violent patients, and injuries caused by traffic accidents involving ambulances. As a consequence, the rate of work-related fatalities among EMS personnel is more than two times higher than that for the general public.

To reduce this danger the Department of Homeland Security (DHS) has collaborated with the National Institute of Standards and Technology (NIST), the National Institute of Occupational Safety and Health (NIOSH), and BMT Designers and Planners in a new ambulance design research. The findings of this effort will be a set of recommendations for incorporation into the next draft (2013) of the National Fire Protection Agency (NFPA) 1917 standard. The results should enhance the physical layout of the ambulance patient compartment and also address broader human factors and human performance issues once the necessary research, development, and testing are completed.

The very first step of NIST's ambulance standard project is to perform a literature survey. A lot of research has already been conducted in ambulance design and is found in disparate locations. Thus the purpose of this report is to provide an annotated bibliography of the literature for a quick, single-source reference for the researchers who are studying the same or related research topic.

2. OVERVIEW OF THE REPORT

This report is a compilation of research that has been done on the ambulance design with the focus on safety and performance in the patient compartment of ambulances, especially for emergency medical technicians, paramedics, and patients. This report is a collection of standards and documents from standard development organizations, journals, websites, and conference proceedings. There are more than eighty papers included in this report. The author(s), title, journal, volume, page(s), publisher, date, and other referential information are noted in the bibliographical annotation. An abstract and parts of the article directly copied from contents of its complimentary referenced document is marked with an asterisk, (*).

The categorization set for this is to make searching the paper in particular topics an easier task for researchers. The major categories that have been identified for the purpose include:

- Ambulance Problems Awareness: Gives background idea behind the types of problems and issues that emergency medical services personnel face from working in their ambulances.
- Injury & Accident Reports: Includes statistics or reports that involve ambulance injuries, fatalities, and accidents.
- Layout & Space Design: Consists of studies conducted to survey and evaluate the space and layout of the ambulance patient compartment.
- Crash Test Procedures: Puts together a few sources that have critiqued and analyzed current ambulance crash test procedures, with suggestions for progress in this field.
- Other Research & Proposed Solutions: Consists of sources that have not been categorized in any other categories, and they include literature about surveys, exterior conspicuity, and more.
- Overall Design Evaluations and Examples: Incorporates surveys and evaluations that have been conducted in order to look at major design problems inside an ambulance. It also includes a few newer design concepts that have been presented by manufacturers.
- Securing People & Equipment: Deals with various restraint systems that are used in ambulances.
- Standards & Guidelines: Reviews national and international ambulance standards and guidelines.

In some instances, these categories do overlap.

3. BIBLIOGRAPHY

3.1 Ambulance Problems Awareness

About.com. "The Difference Between an EMT and a Paramedic." Accessed July 15, 2011. http://firstaid.about.com/od/emergencymedicalservices/qt/06_EMTBvsP.htm.

ABSTRACT: This paper describes the differences among different emergency medical technician (EMT) levels: EMT-Basic, EMT-Intermediate, and EMT-Paramedic. The biggest difference between paramedics and EMTs is in the tasks they are allowed to perform. Also, the amount of training they receive is different. Basic EMTs receive about 120 to 150 hours of training while paramedics receive around 1200-1800 hours of training. In most states, Basic EMTs do not have the privilege to give injections to the patient. Paramedics are usually trained to use 30-40 different medications and are trained to give injections. Ambulance crew members are expected to be at least an EMT-Basic.

Center for Disease Control - National Institute of Occupational Safety and Health. "A Story of Impact: NIOSH Research Leads to a Reduction in Safety Hazards Among Ambulance Service Workers and EMS Responders." Accessed July 18, 2011. http://www.cdc.gov/niosh/docs/2010-164/.

ABSTRACT: In 2006, there was an estimated 201000 emergency medical technician (EMT) and paramedics workforce and at least 700000 volunteer EMTs. Unfortunately, in 2002 it was found that the fatality rate among this workforce was greater than 2 times the national average for workers. Thus, the National Occupational Research Agenda, along with the National Institute of Occupational Safety and Health, set out a mission to evaluate and find any risk factors that are associated with the integrity of the ambulance structure, layout, and human and mechanical barriers. These evaluations and findings will in turn help with revising the federal ambulance standards, which is being done in conjunction with the Ambulance Manufacturers Division (AMD) and the General Services Administration.

Cook, R.I., M. Render, and D.D. Woods. "Gaps in the continuity of care and progress on patient safety." British Medical Journal, 2000, 320: pp 791-794.
*ABSTRACT: The patient safety movement includes a wide variety of approaches and views about how to characterise patient safety, study failure and success, and improve safety. Ultimately all these approaches make reference to the nature of technical work of practitioners at the "sharp end" in the complex, rapidly changing, and intrinsically hazardous world of health care. It is clear that a major activity of technical workers (physicians, nurses, technicians, pharmacists, and others) is coping with complexity and, in particular, coping with the gaps that complexity spawns. Exploration of gaps and the way practitioners anticipate, detect, and bridge them is a fruitful means of pursuing robust improvements in patient safety.

Elling, R. "Dispelling Myths on Ambulance Accidents." Journal of Emergency Medical Services, July 1989.
*ABSTRACT: There appears to be a self-perpetuating trail of misinformation surrounding the issue of ambulance accidents. As with all problems, we must first acknowledge that a problem does exist and clearly distinguish the facts from the myths. The intent of this article was to clarify some of those misconceptions by using an analysis of one state's four-year experience with ambulance accidents. The next step in solving this problem is to create driver education programs that modify the behavior of ambulance drivers, adjust their attitudes about driving an emergency vehicle and make them fully aware of the hazards encountered in driving an ambulance. In addition, consider adjusting the agency standard operating procedure so that all ambulances must come to a complete stop at all stop signs and red lights to minimize the number of accidents that occur in the intersection. Readers who would like to learn more about this subject should contact their state EMS offices to determine if they offer emergency vehicle operator courses or continuing education programs that deal with ambulance driving. New York State has developed a network of 90 instructors who are qualified to teach the Ambulance Accident Prevention Seminar, a nine-hour classroom-based ambulance driver "attitude adjustment" program. Two other organizations that have developed driving courses geared specifically for ambulance driving are: Failsafe Driving Inc. Alvin F. Davenport, president 2529 San Pablo Ave. Pinole, CA 94564 National Academy for Professional Driving Dick Turner, chairman 1001-A South Interstate 45 P.O. Box 649 Hutchins, TX 75141.

Thompson, J. "Ambulance transports safety standards a 'disgrace,' EMS Expo told." Accessed August 17, 2011. http://www.ems1.com/safety/articles/886729-CareFlite-CEO-calls-transport-safety-standards-a-disgrace/.
ABSTRACT: An EMS Expo session was told that the U.S has more safety standards in place for the transport of cattle than for the transport of prehospital care providers and patients. Measures that have been proved to reduce risk, according to the CareFlite CEO Jim Swartz, include: Vehicle operations safety policies, squad bench lap seat belts, patient over the shoulder harnesses, securing equipment, forward and rear facing seating, some electronic technical devices, and safety awareness.

Finkelstein, A., and J.A. Dowell. "A comedy of errors: The London Ambulance Service case study." Paper presented at the proceedings of the 8th International Workshop on Software Specification and Design, Schloss Velen, Germany, March 22-23, 1996.
*ABSTRACT: This paper provides an introduction to the IWSSD-8 case study - the "Report of the Inquiry into the London Ambulance Service". The paper gives an overview of the case study and provides a brief summary. It considers how the case study can be used to orient discussion at the workshop and provide a bridge between the various contributions.

Levick, N. "Rig Safety 911: What You Need to Know About Ambulance Safety and Standards." Journal of Emergency Medical Services, October 2008: pp 66-67.
ABSTRACT: This article highlights the absence of meaningful, scientific-based federal standards for ambulance patient compartments. It also discusses challenges and recommendations to identify best practices in vehicle safety, and new developments in vehicles, technology, policies, and standards that will save lives, time, and money. The article identifies the lack of intrusion testing on current standards.

Louis-Smith, E. "Human engineering concerns in ambulance interior design." Human Factors and Ergonomics Society Annual Meeting Proceedings, 1986, 30(4): pp 345-348.
*ABSTRACT: Although federal specifications do exist and are strictly applied, (Fed. Spec KKK-A-1822) sources of inefficiency and hazard still result in interior ambulance design. Since the "ultimate" ambulance design is not yet a reality and most departments cannot afford to modify everything they please it was considered important to set certain priorities concerning the design of ambulance interiors.

Middleman, S. "Considerations in Medical Ground Transportation." The Case Manager, 2004.
*ABSTRACT: Physicians and nurses, therapists and specialists, case managers and patients and families each form a piece of the health care puzzle. Each party plays a vital role in patient wellness, but if patients do not or cannot get to therapy, they cannot be expected to get better. Patient transportation is improving because case managers can ensure that they have proper transportation to get to appointments locally and out of town.

Slattery, D.E., and A. Silver. "The Hazards of Providing Care in Emergency Vehicles: An Opportunity for Reform." Pre-hospital Emergency Care, 2009, 13(3): pp 388-397.
*ABSTRACT: The risk of occupational death is disproportionately high for emergency medical services (EMS) personnel, largely as a consequence of the high incidence of transportation-related fatalities. The purpose of this narrative review is twofold: to raise awareness in the EMS community by examining the various factors that contribute to vehicular EMS injuries and fatalities and to outline practical strategies for mitigating these risks to EMS professionals. This review describes three main categories of factors that contribute to personnel risk during ambulance transport: the inherent risks of driving/riding in an ambulance, poor ambulance safety standards and design, and increased provider vulnerability to injury while delivering critical patient care in the back of a moving ambulance. Specific educational, technologic, regulatory, and behavioral

strategies for mitigating these risks are offered in hopes of improving ambulance safety practices.

Studnek, J.R., A. Ferketich, and J.M. Crawford. "On the job illness and injury resulting in lost work time among a national cohort of emergency medical services professionals." American journal of industrial medicine 2007, 50(12): pp 921-931. Accessed July 15, 2011.

*ABSTRACT: Background: The objective of this study was to estimate the prevalence and incidence of job-related illness or injury resulting in lost work time among a national cohort of Emergency Medical Services (EMS) professionals. Also, it was hypothesized that individual and work life characteristics were associated with the occurrence of illnesses or injury. Methods: Data for this analysis were obtained from the Longitudinal Emergency Medical Technician Attributes and Demographics Study (LEADS), a prospective study of EMS professionals. The outcome variable of interest was self-reported absence from their EMS job due to an EMS work related illness or injury. The prevalence and incidence of injury with lost work time was estimated using cross-sectional and follow-up data. Multivariable logistic regression analyses were performed to determine if individual and work life characteristics were associated with occupational injury. Results: The prevalence of job-related illness or injury with time away from work was estimated at 9.4 %, while the 1-year incidence was estimated at 8.1 per 100 EMS providers. The results from the logistic regression model fit to follow-up data indicate that increasing call volume (OR=3.12 for very high vs. moderate, 95 % CI 1.40-6.97), an urban work environment (OR=2.79, 95 % CI 1.65-4.72) and a history of back problems (OR=1.72, 95 % CI 1.06-2.78) were associated with reporting job-related illness or injury. Conclusions: Results from this analysis provide estimates of the prevalence and incidence of on the job illness and injury resulting in lost work time among a national cohort of EMS professionals.

3.2 Injury & Accident Reports

Auerbach, P.S., J.A. Jr. Morris, J.B. Jr. Phillips, S.R. Redlinger, and W.K. Vaughn. "An Analysis of Ambulance Accidents in Tennessee." The Journal of the American Medical Association, 1987, 258: pp 1487-1490.
*ABSTRACT: In an effort to improve our program for ambulance crash and related injury prevention, we analyzed 102 consecutive ambulance accidents. Incidents reported included those that resulted in human injury or in which property damage exceeded $200. Multiple logistic regression was used to determine the association between circumstances reported at the time of the accidents and the risk of injury. Twenty-nine accidents contributed to a total of 65 injured victims, with one death. The variable most strongly associated with the probability of an injury-accident was use of a passenger restraint device. Darkness and occurrence at an intersection were variables showing increased risk, but were not statistically significant. The interaction of variables did not have a combined influence on the incidence of injury. The mean delay to hospital care after an accident was 9.4 minutes. Based on our data, we conclude that passenger restraints for both ambulance attendants and passengers should be mandatory, and we suggest that traffic signals be strictly heeded at intersections and speed limits in urban settings be obeyed.

Ballam, E. "Ambulance Crash Roundup: A Review of Emergency Vehicle Crashes During 2010." EMS World, March 2011, 40(3): pp 74-75.
ABSTRACT: A roundup of ambulance crashes that made the news tells us that 264 ambulance-related crashes occurred in the United States, although it is likely that there were even more collisions as there are around 50,000 ambulances on duty on any given day. Of these crashes, 43 % occur where two or more roads cross, and which in the bulk of this 43 % the ambulances were hit by vehicles as they attempted to go through the intersection. Apart from intersection controls, which is the largest factor in these crashes, about 10 % of these crashes appeared to come from the loss of control of the ambulances. Another crash factor road conditions, especially icy and snowy conditions, made up for at least 20 of these crash cases. 21 of the 264 crashes came from rear-end collisions, no fewer than 16 was connected to drug/alcohol abuse, and moose, deer, debris, and rairlroad crossing gates contributed to a few more of the crashes. Furthermore, at least 10 of these collisions involved another ambulance. Reviewing these reported statistics tells us that ambulances are especially prone to danger at intersections. In scenarios involving the ambulances to cross an intersection, slowing down and watching out for changing road conditions may save lives.

EMS World. "Ambulance Crashes: Fatality Factors for EMS Workers." Accessed July 19, 2011. http://www.emsworld.com/print/EMS-World/Ambulance-Crashes--Fatality-Factors-for-EMS-Workers/1$1796.
ABSTRACT: In the Morbidity and Mortality Weekly Report article published in

February 2003, the National Institute for Occupational Safety and Health (NIOSH) identified 27 EMS worker fatalities. These fatalities were a result of ambulance crashes reported to the National Highway Traffic Safety Administration's Fatality Analysis Reporting System (FARS) for the years 1991-2000. This article presents a more in-depth look at the 25 crashes that resulted in these 27 fatalities, focusing primarily on ambulance configurations, roadway and environmental conditions, and driver-related factors. A key finding was that weather and road conditions did not appear to play significant roles in most crashes, but driving the ambulance too fast and/or in the wrong lane were notable factors. Another interesting characteristic of these fatality factors was that nearly half of the ambulance drivers in all of the fatal crashes had some kind of collision/moving driving violation within 3 years of the fatal event.

Kahn, C.A., R.G. Pirallo, and E.M. Kuhn. "Characteristics of fatal ambulance crashes in the United States: an 11-year retrospective analysis."
Prehospital Emergency Care: The Official Journal of the National Association of EMS Physicians and the National Association of State EMS Directors, 2001, 5(3): pp 261-269. Accessed July 15, 2011.
*ABSTRACT: Background: Ambulance crashes have become an increasing source of public concern. Emergency medical services directors have little data to develop ambulance operation and risk management policies. Objective: This paper describes fatal ambulance crash characteristics, identifying those that differentiate emergency and non-emergency use crashes. Mehods: This was a retrospective analysis of all fatal ambulance crashes on U.S. public roadways reported to the Fatality Analysis Reporting System (FARS) database from 1987 to 1997. Main outcome measures were 42 variables describing crash demographics, crash configuration, vehicle description, crash severity, and ambulance operator and vehicle occupant attributes. Results: Three hundred thirty-nine ambulance crashes caused 405 fatalities and 838 injuries. These crashes occurred more often between noon and 6 PM (39 %), on improved (99 %), straight (86 %), dry roads (69 %) during clear weather (77 %), while going straight (80 %), through an intersection (53 %), and striking (81 %) another vehicle (80 %) at an angle (56 %). Most crashes (202/339) and fatalities (233/405) occurred during emergency use. These crashes occurred significantly more often at intersections ($p < 0.001$), at an angle ($p < 0.001$), with another vehicle ($p < 0.001$). Most crashes resulted in one fatality, not in the ambulance. Thirty pedestrians and one bicyclist comprised 9 % of all fatalities. In the ambulance, most serious and fatal injuries occurred in the rear (OR 2.7 vs. front) and to improperly restrained occupants (OR 2.5 vs. restrained). Sixteen percent of ambulance operators were cited; 41 % had poor driving records. Conclusions: Most crashes and fatalities occurred during emergency use and at intersections. The greater burden of injury fell upon persons not in the ambulance. Rear compartment occupants were more likely to be injured than those in the front. Crash and injury reduction programs should address improved intersection control, screening to identify high-risk drivers, appropriate restraint use, and design modifications to the rear compartment of the ambulance.

Lutman, D., M. Montgomery, P. Ramnarayan, and A. Petros. "Ambulance and aeromedical accident rates during emergency retrieval in Great Britain." **Emergency Medicine Journal**, 2008, 25: pp 301-302. Accessed on July 25, 2011. doi: 10.1136/emj.2007.046557.
*ABSTRACT: The retrieval of critically ill patients is frequently done in difficult circumstances and often under considerable time pressures. These adverse conditions have a finite risk of serious injury or death. The level of risk is poorly described in the literature and reliable data on accident rates are hard to find. Most of the information comes from North America. There are no clear published statistics for the UK. We report for the first time data on accidents and casualties involving vehicles classified as having an ambulance body type and air ambulances within Great Britain between 1999 and 2004.

Maguire, B.J., K.L. Hunting, G.S. Smith, and N.R. Levick. "Occupational Fatalities in Emergency Medical Services: A Hidden Crisis." **Annals of Emergency Medicine**, 2002, 40(6): pp 625-632.
*ABSTRACT: Study Objective: We estimate the occupational fatality rate among emergency medical services (EMS) personnel in the United States. Methods: We undertook descriptive epidemiology of occupational fatalities among EMS providers. Analysis was conducted by using data from 3 independent fatality databases: the Census of Fatal Occupational Injuries (1992 to 1997), the National EMS Memorial Service (1992 to 1997), and the National Highway Traffic Safety Administration's Fatality Analysis Reporting System (1994 to 1997). These rates were compared with the occupational fatality rates of police and firefighters and with the rate of all employed persons in the United States. Results: The Census of Fatal Occupational Injuries database documented 91 EMS provider occupational fatalities. The National EMS Memorial Service database contained 70 fatalities, and the Fatality Analysis Reporting System identified 8 ground-transportation EMS occupational fatalities. There was also wide variation in fatality counts by cause of injury. Using the highest cause-specific count from each of the databases, we estimate that there were at least 67 ground transportation-related fatalities, 19 air ambulance crash fatalities, 13 deaths resulting from cardiovascular incidents, 10 homicides, and 5 other causes, resulting in 114 EMS worker fatalities during these 6 years. We estimated a rate of 12.7 fatalities per 100,000 EMS workers annually, which compares with 14.2 for police, 16.5 for firefighters, and a national average of 5.0 during the same time period. Conclusion: This study identifies an occupational fatality rate for EMS workers that exceeds that of the general population and is comparable with that of other emergency public service workers.

Proudfoot, S.L., P. Moore, and R. Levine. "Safety In Numbers: A Survey on Ambulance Patient Compartment Safety." **Journal of Emergency Medical Services,** March 2007, 32(3): pp 86-90.

ABSTRACT: A study in 2004 was conducted by the National Registry of EMTs (NREMT) and the National Highway Traffic Safety Administration (NHTSA) in order to identify safety issues related to the ambulance patient compartment. In this study, 1773 EMTs and paramedics responded to a questionnaire. 55 % of the respondents said that they would use patient compartment restraints if they allowed mobility, while 23 % said they will rarely wear such restraints. 29 % said they would wear a helmet with integrated communications system, while 49 % said they will rarely wear the helmet. Over 66 % have transported 2 or more patients within the past year, and only 26 % of them have ever used the defibrillator. The results of this study showed that, in order to increase safety measures in the ambulance patient compartment, providers and equipment within the ambulance should always be secured or fastened. Also, when transporting patients, the EMTs or paramedics must sit in a side-facing or rear-facing position. In general, the findings from this study shows an increasing need to research better seating and equipment location and security, as well as mobile restraint systems.

Proudfoot, S.L., N.T. Romano, T.G. Bobick, and P.H. Moore. "Ambulance crash-related injuries among emergency medical services workers - United States, 1991-2002." Journal of the American Medical Association, April 2003, 289(13): pp 1628-1629.
*ABSTRACT: Ambulance crashes are one of many hazards faced by Emergency Medical Services (EMS) personnel. Although no complete national count of ground ambulance crashes exists, the total number of fatal crashes involving ambulances can be ascertained by using the National Highway Traffic Safety Administration (NHTSA) Fatality Analysis Reporting System (FARS). To characterize risk factors for EMS workers involved in ambulance crashes, CDC's National Institute for Occupational Safety and Health (NIOSH) and NHTSA investigated three case reports of ambulance crashes. This report summarizes these investigations, presents surveillance data, and discusses recommendations for prevention measures. NIOSH is identifying and testing alternative measures to reduce injury risk for EMS workers.

Ray, A.M, and D.F. Kupas. "Comparison of Rural and Urban Ambulance Crashes in Pennsylvania." Prehospital Emergency Care, 2007, 11(4): pp 416-422.
*ABSTRACT: Objective: To describe and compare the characteristics of, and associated injuries caused by, ambulance crashes that occur in rural versus urban areas. Methods: Crash data collected by the Pennsylvania Department of Transportation were obtained for ambulance crashes from 1997 to 2001. Crash demographics (e.g., location of crash, road conditions, and intersection type) and injuries reported by police were analyzed to determine differences, if any, between crashes occurring in rural and urban areas. Results: 311 rural and 1,434 urban ambulance crashes were identified. Day and time of crash, light conditions

and road type were similar. Rural crashes were more likely to occur on snowy roads (13 % vs. 5 %) and at nighttime without street lighting (25 % vs. 4 %). Operator error was the most common cause of crashes (75 % for rural; 93 % for urban), whereas vehicle or environmental conditions more frequently affected rural drivers (25 % vs. 7 %). Urban crashes were more likely to involve angled collisions with other vehicles (54 % vs. 19 %), intersections (67 % vs. 26 %), and occur at a stop sign or signal (53 % vs. 14 %). Rural crashes often involved striking a fixed object (33 % vs. 7 %). Urban crashes more often involved more than one vehicle (88 % vs. 56 %) and more than four people total (35 % vs. 23 %). Pedestrian involvement was rare in both groups (<5 %). Injury severity was similar between both types of crashes, although rural crashes more frequently did not involve any injuries (33 % vs. 20 %). Alcohol and/or drug use by drivers was rare (<1 %). Conclusion: Rural ambulance crashes usually do not involve other vehicles and are more often due to environmental or vehicle factors. Urban ambulance crashes typically involve intersections, other vehicles, and traffic signals. Although more people and vehicles are often involved in urban ambulance crashes, the severity of injuries sustained are similar.

Reichard, A.A., and L.L. Jackson. "Occupational Injuries Among Emergency Responders." American Journal of Industrial Medicine, 2009: pp 1-11.
*ABSTRACT: Background: Emergency responders frequently incur injuries while providing medical, fire, and law enforcement services. National surveillance systems provide fragmented perspectives on responder injuries because they omit specific classes of workers (e.g., government or volunteers); they report only selected injuries; and employment information is incomplete. Methods: We characterized injuries among emergency medical services (EMS), firefighting, and police occupations by using data from the National Electronic Injury Surveillance System-Occupational Supplement (NEISS-Work) for injuries treated in U.S. hospital emergency departments in 2000-2001. Results: Sprains and strains were the leading injury (33 to 41%) among EMS, firefighter, and police occupations. Police officers and career firefighters had the highest injury rates (8.5 and 7.4 injuries per 100 full-time equivalent workers, respectively). Conclusions: The physical demands of emergency response are a leading cause of injuries that may benefit from similar interventions across the occupations. To assess risk, improved exposure data need to be acquired, particularly for volunteers.

Sanddal, N.D., S. Albert, J.D. Hansen, and D.F. Kupas. "Contributing factors and issues associated with rural ambulance crashes: literature review and annotated bibliography." Prehospital Emergency Care, 2008, 12(2): pp 257-267.
*ABSTRACT: Ambulance crashes occur with greater frequency and severity than crashes involving vehicles of similar size and weight characteristics. Crashes in rural areas tend to be more severe in terms of injury or death to vehicle

occupants. The purpose of this article was to examine the extant literature, as well as summarize and discuss the overlapping findings of that body of literature. A stepwise literature search was conducted using the following MeSH search terms ambulance; accident, traffic; emergency medical technician; occupational health; and rural in descending combination. MEDLINE was used as the primary database but was augmented by searches of Academic Search Premier, Comprehensive Index of Nursing, Allied Health Literature, and ProQuest Dissertation International. The search resulted in 32 article citations, and of these, 28 were included. An annotated bibliography is followed by a discussion and conclusion that identify opportunities for prevention activities in the areas of education, enforcement, and engineering.

Sanddal, T.L, N.D. Sanddal, N. Ward, and L. Stanley. "Ambulance Crash Characteristics in the US Defined by the Popular Press: A Retrospective Analysis." Emergency Medicine International, 2010: 7 pages. Accessed July 14, 2011. doi: 10.1155/2010/525979.
*ABSTRACT: Ambulance crashes are a significant risk to prehospital care providers, the patients they are carrying, persons in other vehicles, and pedestrians. No uniform national transportation or medical database captures all ambulance crashes in the United States. A website captures many significant ambulance crashes by collecting reports in the popular media (the website is mentioned in the introduction). This report summarizes findings from ambulance crashes for the time period of May 1, 2007 to April 30, 2009. Of the 466 crashes examined, 358 resulted in injuries to prehospital personnel, other vehicle occupants, patients being transported in the ambulance, or pedestrians. A total of 982 persons were injured as a result of ambulance crashes during the time period. Prehospital personnel were the most likely to be injured. Provider safety can and should be improved by ambulance vehicle redesign and the development of improved occupant safety restraints. Seventy-nine (79) crashes resulted in fatalities to some member of the same groups listed above. A total of 99 persons were killed in ambulance crashes during the time period. Persons in other vehicles involved in collisions with ambulances were the most likely to die as a result of crashes. In the urban environment, intersections are a particularly dangerous place for ambulances.

Studnek, J.R., and A.R. Fernandez. "Characteristics of emergency medical technicians involved in ambulance crashes." Prehospital Disaster Medicine, 2008, 23(5): pp 432-437.
*ABSTRACT: Objectives: This study utilizes a [US] national sample of emergency medical services (EMS) professionals to explore the hypothesis that demographic and work-related characteristics are associated with involvement in ambulance crashes. Methods: In 2004, a cohort of nationally registered EMS professionals was surveyed to determine ambulance crash involvement during a 12-month period. Involvement in an ambulance crash was the outcome variable of interest. Demographics such as age, community size, service type, call

volume, time spent in an ambulance, and current sleep problems were analyzed as independent variables. A multivariate logistic regression model identified variables associated with involvement in an ambulance crash within the past year. Results: Surveys were received from 1775/5565 (32.0 %) participants; 1297 (73.1 %) met the inclusion criteria. A total of 111 (8.6 %) of participants reported being involved in an ambulance crash within the past 12 months. When controlling for call volume and time in an ambulance, the odds of involvement in an ambulance crash within the past year were significantly higher for younger EMS professionals and those reporting sleep problems. Conclusions: Results from this analysis suggest age and sleep problems are associated with involvement in an ambulance crash. Future studies should investigate interventions to minimize the effects of these associations.

Tetreault, M.W. "Evaluating Injuries to Firefighters While Performing Patient Care in a Moving Ambulance." An applied research project submitted to the National Fire Academy as part of the Executive Officer Program, Londonderry, New Hampshire, May 2009.

*ABSTRACT: The Londonderry firefighters and their equipment are not properly restrained while performing patient care in the back of a moving ambulance. In the event of a crash the firefighter or the patient could be injured or killed due to this uncontrolled movement of personnel and equipment. This research is to evaluate the types and mechanisms of injuries to passengers in the back of a moving ambulance and to determine which methods are most effective in preventing such injuries. The purpose of this research is to prevent injury and death to firefighters and patients be transported in an ambulance. The descriptive research method was used to answer the following relevant questions: (1) What are the current mechanisms for preventing uncontrolled movement of firefighters while caring for patients in a moving ambulance? (2) What are the types and mechanisms of injury that occur to firefighters while riding in the patient compartment of a moving ambulance? (3) What strategies would have been successful in preventing uncontrolled movement during patient care, and how have these affected patient care? (4) What modifications can be made from technological and/or procedural perspective to decrease the effects of uncontrolled movement of firefighters riding in the patient compartment of a moving ambulance? The results focused upon necessary policy modifications, and the technological modifications needed for current in-service ambulances, current ambulance purchases and what to expect in the future. Finally advocating for comprehensive crash worthiness standards for ambulances including, federal oversight and crash testing to determine what changes need to be made in ambulance design.

3.3 Layout & Space Design

Alejo, J.S., M.G. Martin, M. Ortega-Mier, and A. Garcia-Sanchez. "Mixed integer programming model for optimizing the layout of an ICU vehicle." BMC Health Services Research, 2009, 9(224): pp 1-14. Accessed July 21, 2011. doi: 10.1186/1472-6963-9-224.

*ABSTRACT: Background: This paper presents a Mixed Integer Programming (MIP) model for designing the layout of the Intensive Care Units' (ICUs) patient care space. In particular, this MIP model was developed for optimizing the layout for materials to be used in interventions. This work was developed within the framework of a joint project between the Madrid Technical University and the Medical Emergency Services of the Madrid Regional Government (SUMMA 112). Methods: The first task was to identify the relevant information to define the characteristics of the new vehicles and, in particular, to obtain a satisfactory interior layout to locate all the necessary materials. This information was gathered from health workers related to ICUs. With that information, an optimization model was developed in order to obtain a solution. From the MIP model, a first solution was obtained, consisting of a grid to locate the different materials needed for the ICUs. The outcome from the MIP model was discussed with health workers to tune the solution, and after slightly altering that solution to meet some requirements that had not been included in the mathematical model, the eventual solution was approved by the persons responsible for specifying the characteristics of the new vehicles. According to the opinion stated by the SUMMA 112's medical group responsible for improving the ambulances (the so-called "coaching group"), the outcome was highly satisfactory. Indeed, the final design served as a basis to draw up the requirements of a public tender. Results: As a result from solving the Optimization model, a grid was obtained to locate the different necessary materials for the ICUs. This grid had to be slightly altered to meet some requirements that had not been included in the mathematical model. The results were discussed with the persons responsible for specifying the characteristics of the new vehicles. Conclusion: The outcome was highly satisfactory. Indeed, the final design served as a basis to draw up the requirements of a public tender. The authors advocate this approach to address similar problems within the field of Health Services to improve the efficiency and the effectiveness of the processes involved. Problems such as those in operation rooms or emergency rooms, where the availability of a large amount of material is critical are eligible to be dealt with in a similar manner.

Ferreira, J., and S. Hignett. "Reviewing ambulance design for clinical efficiency and paramedic safety." Applied Ergonomics, 2005, 36: pp 97-105.
*ABSTRACT: This study aimed to review the layout of the patient compartment in a UK ambulance for paramedic efficiency and safety using: (1) link analysis; (2) postural analysis. Paramedics were observed over 16 shifts (130 hours) carrying out a range of clinical tasks. The most frequently occurring clinical tasks were

checking blood oxygen saturation, oxygen administration, monitoring the heart and checking blood pressure. Access to the equipment and consumables to support these tasks had been designed for the attendant seat (head end of the stretcher), however, a link analysis found that paramedics preferred to sit along side the stretcher which resulted in increased reach distances. The higher frequency tasks were found to include over 40 % of working postures which required corrective measures. It was concluded that future ambulance design should be based on an ergonomics analysis (including link analysis and postural analysis) of clinical activities.

Gilad, I., and E. Byran. "Ergonomic Evaluation of the Ambulance Interior to Reduce Paramedic Discomfort and Posture Stress." Human Factors, 2007, 49, pp 1019-1032.
*ABSTRACT: OBJECTIVE: This study aims to evaluate safety and accessibility of an advanced life support (ALS) ambulance interior. BACKGROUND: The standard ambulance's interior design is unsatisfactory based on perceived discomfort and postures that constrain paramedics and medical staff, resulting in unsafe treatment of patients, mainly when being transported. METHODS: Two procedures were used to evaluate performance during a wide range of rescue tasks: a survey, based on questionnaires, interviews, and observation of paramedics performing routine tasks; and upper body and back posture analysis, based on postural considerations. RESULTS: Findings revealed that 74 % of the paramedics stated that the location of the paramedic's seat is inefficient while they perform clinical procedures; 94 % found the bench uncomfortable; 77 % felt that the vertical distance between the bench and the stretcher is too far; and 86% needed to steady themselves when the vehicle was moving. Posture analysis showed that paramedics undergo several non-neutral back postures, including twisted back (>20°) and sitting with back flexion between 20 degrees and 45 degrees. CONCLUSION: Because the interior of the ALS ambulance was found to be unsatisfactory both to paramedics and patients, alternative design issues are proposed. APPLICATION: The suggested practical layout contains four main modifications: (a) replacing the bench with two adjustable paramedic seats, (b) redesigning the medical cabinet for easy access, (c) adding an adjustable folding seat opposite the two new seats, and (d) adding a swiveling base and lifting apparatus that will accommodate the stretcher and enable better accessibility to patients by the paramedic personnel.

Mueller, J. "Naturalistic data collection in rural emergency medical services transportation." Paper presented at the annual national rural IIT Conference Student Paper Competition, 2010.
*ABSTRACT: This paper examines the behaviors of emergency medical service (EMS) workers during emergency medical transport. The study uses an advanced naturalistic data collection system to record visual, vehicle, and accessory parameters associated with each ambulance trip. Visual data was analyzed to look at restraint characteristics, position within the ambulance data,

and posture data to identify areas where medics are subject to poor working conditions.

Safar, P., and R.A. Brose. "Ambulance Design and Equipment for Resuscitation." Archives of Surgery, 1965, 30(3): pp 343-348.
ABSTRACT: Improved emergency care for the critically ill or injured physician leadership in community-wide teaching and organization of (1) first aid; (2) ambulance transportation; and (3) hospital emergency room coverage. Airway obstruction, respiratory depression, and cardiac arrest from unconsciousness per se (e.g., head injury, poisoning) and from such conditions as drowning, coronary occlusion, electric shock, and others can often be prevented or reversed if the rescuer is trained in the proper techniques, begins resuscitation immediately, and continues resuscitation during transportation to the hospital. Modern inhalation therapy and resuscitation during transportation are often hampered by inadequate design and equipment. Personal experience with the deficiencies of existing ambulance design, experience with many resuscitations outside of ambulances, established principles of resuscitation, and successful use of some of the modifications recommended prompted us to write this paper. Locally, appropriate modifications were made on a model ambulance, which was used during the first nine months in 21 calls. Suction was used 4 times; oxygen, 31 times; and bag-mask ventilation, 19 times, all satisfactorily. In addition, the new equipment was used successfully during manikin practice in the moving ambulance.

Sanchez, F.J., A. Garcia-Sanchez, M. Ortega-Mier, and J.M. Lopez. "Design of the patient care space inside an ICU vehicle or ambulance through an optimization model." International Journal of Heavy Vehicle Systems, 2010, 17(1): pp 35-51.
*ABSTRACT: The primary results of a project aimed at improving interior patient care space design of Madrid (Spain) regional government medical emergency services intensive care units in vehicles such as ambulances are presented. To carry out the study, researchers gathered data and criteria from health workers, from which they developed an optimization model. This model allowed them to obtain a solution as to how to locate all medical health materials and equipment so that the more critical and frequent operations could be performed. These operations needed to be done in with shortest possible time, without interfering with the efforts of health care workers and with materials as close as possible to person needing the equipment.

Snook, R. "Medical Aspects of Ambulance Design." British Medical Journal, 1972, 3: pp 574-578.
*ABSTRACT: Various observations have shown that the interior layout of many ambulances leaves much to be desired. The lighting levels are inadequate, heat loss could be prevented, vehicle identification and passage through traffic could be improved, and measurable differences exist between the ride characteristics of commercially available ambulances, a prototype purpose-built ambulance, and

a private car. Moreover the condition of some patients may be affected by the motion of the vehicle either directly or indirectly. Even though they form a small percentage of the total number carried, they represent a very considerable financial risk. A personally conducted survey of ambulance chief officers showed a deep interest and involvement in the upgrading of the service with a general dissatisfaction with many of the vehicles currently available. Hence there is a market for the purpose-built ambulance, which would benefit the patient and the ambulanceman alike.

The inadequacies of many vehicles currently in use as ambulances have been shown to work against the interests of the patient requiring life support treatment, and it is suggested that this warrants urgent attention and action. A more extensive research project involving medical observations on the supine sick and injured, attendant task performance, and instrumentation analysis of linear and angular vehicle motions should enable the harmful effects of ride motion to be identified.

None of these investigations, however, will be of any value unless they are used in developing future ambulances. Such development must also parallel an increase in the awareness of the importance of ambulance design and its relation to the increased comfort and chance of survival of the patients carried.

3.4 Crash Test Procedures

Current, R.S., P.H. Moore, J.D. Green, J.R. Yannaccone, G.R. Whitman, and L.A. Sicher. "Crash Testing of Ambulance Chassis Cab Vehicles." Presented at the SAE 2007 Commercial Vehicle Engineering Congress & Exhibition, October 2007.

*ABSTRACT: The National Institute for Occupational Safety and Health (NIOSH), in cooperation with the Canadian Forces Health Services Group Headquarters, U.S. Army Tank-Automotive and Armaments Command (TACOM), and the Ministry of Health & Long-Term Care, Ontario (Canada), conducted a test program to evaluate the capability of mobile restraint systems to protect occupants in the patient compartment of an ambulance. This paper focuses on the vehicle chassis behavior and acceleration pulses as seen in each test conducted to support the program. This program consisted of testing one Type I ambulance mounted on a Ford F-350 truck chassis (1994 vintage), and three Type III ambulances mounted on Ford E-350 van chassis (two 1993, and one 1999 vintage). A vehicle-to-vehicle side impact test was conducted using the Type I ambulance with a targeted change in velocity of 27.4 kph (17 mph). A 1984 Chevrolet Sierra 2500 was the impacting vehicle for the side test. Fixed barrier frontal tests were conducted using the Type III ambulances with a targeted impact velocity of 48 kph (30 mph). In addition to an x-axis, or forward component, each of the frontal crash pulses was found to have a significant z-axis, or vertical, component which caused a forward rotation of the patient compartment ranging up to approximately 16.5 degrees. Significant cab-intrusion was observed as a result of the frontal tests that were conducted. Vehicle weights ranged up to 5005 kg (11,035 lbs.) and were similar to operational weight conditions. The paper includes a detailed description of the crash test setup as it pertains to the chassis, vehicles tested, instrumentation, limited crush measurements, testing observations, and the resulting multi-axial pulses measured at multiple frame and patient compartment locations. This data will be of interest to ambulance and other multi-stage vehicle manufacturers for use in design, modeling, and sled testing.

Levick, N.R., B.R. Donnelly, A. Blatt, G. Gillespie, and M. Schultze. "Ambulance Crashworthiness and Occupant Dynamics in Vehicle-To-Vehicle Crash Tests: Preliminary Report." Paper presented at the proceedings of the 17th International Technical Conference on the Enhanced Safety of Vehicles, Amsterdam, Netherlands, June 2001.

*ABSTRACT: There are no dynamic safety testing standards specifically for ambulance vehicles in the USA. These vehicles have also been identified to have high crash injury and fatality rates per mile, with a majority of the fatalities involving either an intersection or a frontal crash. This study is an interim report on work in progress which demonstrates occupant safety and crashworthiness of ambulance vehicles in vehicle to vehicle intersection type crash tests. The ambulance vehicles were configured with instrumented ATDs (Anthropomorphic

Test Dummies) to represent 95th percentile male, 5th percentile female and 3 year child occupants. A 'real world' configuration of these ATDs and some medical equipment was established for a frontal and side impact crash test. The findings demonstrated life threatening safety hazards for all occupants. Also measured crash pulses for both the vehicle and the interior components were obtained. The urgent need for improvements to ambulance crash safety standards and designs are discussed.

Levick, N.R., and R. Grzebieta. "Development of Proposed Crash Test Procedures for Ambulance Vehicles." Paper presented for Enhanced Safety of Vehicles Conference, Lyon, France, June 18-21, 2007.
*ABSTRACT: Ambulance vehicles are a unique passenger environment with complex crashworthiness and occupant protection issues, e.g. occupants in various orientations, unique human factors aspects and an array of aftermarket interior modifications. In the USA, ambulance vehicle occupant protection, crashworthiness and safety testing lags 30 years behind current general automotive safety technology. This paper proposes crash test procedures and outlines some of the challenges faced for such vehicles based on manufacturer and consumer conducted pre-modification crash tests and previous ambulance sled and full scale crash tests. A typical ambulance vehicle from one of the largest fleets globally, was addressed. Based on manufacturer specifications, crash test data for the vehicle, inspections and other published data regarding ambulance vehicle crashes, sled and crash testing were considered – an approach to an impact testing procedure is outlined and developed by a multidisciplinary team. Assessment and development focused on vehicle crashworthiness performance and real world human factors aspects of aftermarket interior modifications. Frontal and side impact crashworthiness testing profiles for this vehicle were determined and developed inline with parameters outlined in ASA 4535 (ambulance restraint systems standard) and the CEN 1789 standard. The testing profiles include a recumbent occupant, rear and forward facing seated occupants, 50th and 95th percentile ATDs, including side impact ATDs for seating positions exposed to side impacts. The authors propose that ambulance vehicle safety testing and design should be driven by accepted automotive safety practice. In a setting of high crash rates, a complex occupant and emergency care environment, and the absence of prescribed dynamic crashworthiness test procedures for ambulances - the proposed test procedures in this paper provide a first approach to describe the approach to the technical development of comprehensive crash testing profiles in this setting. Such profiles for this environment will ensure that system safety can be ascertained and optimized for these vehicles, and support safety enhancements and occupant protection for ambulance vehicle development.

Levick, N.R., and R. Grzebieta. "USA Ambulance Crashworthiness Frontal Impact Testing." Paper presented at the 21st International Technical Conference on the Enhanced Safety of Vehicles Conference (ESV) - International Congress Center, Stuttgart, Germany, June 15-18, 2009.

*ABSTRACT: Recent epidemiological studies have identified ambulances as high risk passenger transport vehicles, particularly the rear compartment. It appears in the absence of USA ambulance safety standards or guidelines, non engineer end-users are driving changes in practice and policy in place of independent peer reviewed biomechanical and crash injury outcome data. This study's objective is to compare and analyze frontal crash biomechanical and crashworthiness research for ambulance vehicles, with a focus on application of the real world environment, and development needs for future standards. Frontal impact ambulance crashworthiness tests conducted over past 15 years, were identified and evaluated with a multidisciplinary approach consisting of automotive crashworthiness, emergency medicine, public health and EMS care delivery. Crash test data identified include: 25 g-force (gravitational force) to 34 g-force deceleration sled tests (delta V 33.6 km/h (20.9 mph) to 52.0 km/h (32.3 mph)); one full crash test of a bullet vehicle travelling at 57.9 km/h (36 mph) crashing into another vehicle, impact Delta V of 30 km/h (18.5 mph) and deceleration of 14 g-forces to the rear compartment; and three fixed barrier frontal tests at a 40 km/h (25 mph) delta V and 25 g-force impacts. There appeared to be a lack of correlation with real world crash forces in the conduct of the rigid barrier tests. The use of data from side facing occupants was also confounding. Ambulance crashworthiness is a complex system. Clearly demonstrated hazards have been identified in the limited real world crash injury/fatality data and the crash test data available. Testing must be based on meaningful real world parameters such as the forces that occur in actual crashes and the types of injury and fatality hazards to the occupants, so that development of standards and thus the design and construction of ambulance vehicles, can be focused to achieve adequate levels of occupant protection using current crashworthiness methodology already utilized in industry.

3.5 Other Research & Proposed Solutions

Catchpole, K., and D. McKeown. "A framework for the design of ambulance sirens." Ergonomics, 2007, 50(8): pp 1287-1301.
*ABSTRACT: Ambulance sirens are essential for assisting the safe and rapid arrival of an ambulance at the scene of an emergency. In this study, the parameters upon which sirens may be designed were examined and a framework for emergency vehicle siren design was proposed. Validity for the framework was supported through acoustic measurements and the evaluation of ambulance transit times over 240 emergency runs using two different siren systems. Modifying existing siren sounds to add high frequency content would improve vehicle penetration, detectability and sound localization cues, and mounting the siren behind the radiator grill, rather than on the light bar or under the wheel arch, would provide less unwanted noise while maintaining or improving the effective distance in front of the vehicle. Ultimately, these considerations will benefit any new attempt to design auditory warnings for the emergency services.

Cooper, G., and E. Ghassemieh. "Risk assessment of patient handling with ambulance stretcher systems (ramp/(winch), easi-loader, tail-lift) using biomechanical failure criteria." Medical Engineering & Physics, 2007, 29: 775-787.
*ABSTRACT: The research aims to carry out a detailed analysis of the loads applied by the ambulance workers when loading/unloading ambulance stretchers. The forces required of the ambulance workers for each system are measured using a load cell in a force handle arrangement. The process of loading and unloading is video recorded for all the systems to register the posture of the ambulance workers in different stages of the process. The postures and forces exerted by the ambulance workers are analyzed using biomechanical assessment software to examine if the work loads at any stage of the process are harmful. Kinetic analysis of each stretcher loading system is performed. Comparison of the kinetic analysis and measurements shows very close agreement for most of the cases. The force analysis results are evaluated against derived failure criteria. The evaluation is extended to a biomechanical failure analysis of the ambulance worker's lower back using 3DSSPP software developed at the Centre for Ergonomics at the University of Michigan. The critical tasks of each ambulance worker during the loading and unloading operations for each system are identified. Design recommendations are made to reduce the forces exerted based on loading requirements from the kinetic analysis.

Federal Emergency Management Agency. Emergency Vehicle Visibility and Conspicuity Study. FA-323, August 2009.
*ABSTRACT: Over the past decade, numerous law enforcement officers, firefighters, and emergency medical services (EMS) workers were injured or killed along roadways throughout the United States. In 2008, as with the prior 10

years, more law enforcement officers died in traffic-related incidents than from any other cause; National Law Enforcement Officers Memorial (NLEOM, 2008) over the past 12 years, an average of one officer per month was struck and killed by a vehicle in the United States. (FBI, 2007) Preliminary firefighter fatality statistics for 2008 ref lect 29 of 114 firefighters killed on duty perished in motor vehicle crashes, (USFA, 2009a) similar to figures posted in previous years. According to a 2002 study (Maguire, et al.) that aggregated data from several independent sources, at least 67 EMS providers were killed in ground transportation-related events over the 6 years from 1992 to 1997.

These sobering facts clearly demonstrate the importance of addressing vehicle characteristics and human factors for reducing the morbidity and mortality of public safety personnel operating along the Nation's highways and byways. Studies conducted in the United States and elsewhere suggest that increasing emergency vehicle visibility and conspicuity holds promise for enhancing first responders' safety when exposed to traffic both inside and outside their response vehicles (e.g., patrol cars, motorcycles, fire apparatus, and ambulances).

This report, produced in partnership between the U.S. Fire Administration (USFA) and the International Fire Service Training Association (IFSTA), with support from the U.S. Department of Justice (DOJ), National Institute of Justice (NIJ), analyzes emergency vehicle visibility and conspicuity with an eye toward expanding efforts in these areas to improve vehicle and roadway operations safety for all emergency responders. Emphasis in this report is placed on passive visibility/conspicuity treatments; additional studies are underway on active technologies such as emergency vehicle warning lighting systems. (USFA, 2009b)

A number of key findings were developed from the examination performed for this report. Principal among these findings is the salient need for additional research on emergency vehicle visibility and conspicuity in the United States, with particular emphasis on the interaction between civilian drivers and emergency vehicles during responses and on incident scenes.

Despite meaningful limitations, the existing visibility/conspicuity research, combined with passenger vehicle lighting and human factors, evokes several potential opportunities for improving the safety of emergency vehicles in the United States using readily available products.

Hunt, R.C., L.H. Brown, E.S. Cabinum, T.W. Whitley, H. Prasad, C.F. Owens, and C.E. Mayo. "Is ambulance transport time with lights and siren faster than that without?" Annals of Emergency Medicine, 1995, 25(4): pp 507-511.
*ABSTRACT: STUDY OBJECTIVE: To determine whether ambulance transport time from the scene to the emergency department is faster with warning lights and siren than that without. DESIGN: In a convenience sample, transport times and routes of ambulances using lights and sirens were recorded by an observer. The time also was recorded by a paramedic who drove an ambulance without lights and siren over identical routes during simulated transports at the same time of day and on the same day of the week as the corresponding lights-and-siren transport. SETTING: An emergency medical service system in a city with a

population of 46,000. PARTICIPANTS: Emergency medical technicians and paramedics. RESULTS: Fifty transport times with lights and siren averaged 43.5 seconds faster than the transport times without lights and siren [t = 4.21, P = .0001]. CONCLUSION: In this setting, the 43.5 second mean time savings does not warrant the use of lights and siren during ambulance transport, except in rare situations or clinical circumstances.

Jones, A., and S. Hignett. "Safe access/egress systems for emergency ambulances." Emergency Medicine Journal, 2007, 24: pp 200-205. Accessed on July 25, 2011. doi: 10.1136/emj.2006.041707.
*ABSTRACT: OBJECTIVETo comparatively evaluate the three most widely used ambulance stretcher loading systems; easi-loader, ramp/winch and tail lift to identify a preferred system based on safety and usability evidence. METHODS: Three data types were collected in the field, the laboratory and from a national questionnaire. Field data were collected using the qualitative methods of observation (link analysis and hierarchical task analysis) and interview (critical incident technique) over 12 months during 2004–5. Laboratory data were collected for detailed postural analysis. A national ranking questionnaire was used to prioritize the resulting design issues. RESULTS: The field study data were analyzed, triangulated and summarized in a taxonomy to identify the design and operational issues. A list of 14 criteria was used in a national ranking exercise with 134 ambulance staff and manufacturers. Patient and operator safety was ranked as the highest priority, followed by manual handling. The postural analysis found that the easi-loader system presented the highest postural risk. CONCLUSION: The tail lift was found to be the preferred and safest loading system from both the field and laboratory research and is the recommended option from the evaluated loading systems.

Karsh, B.T. "Clinical practice improvement and redesign: how change in workflow can be supported by clinical decision support." Prepared for Agency for Healthcare Research and Quality, Rockville, Maryland, June 2009.
ABSTRACT: Clinical decision support (CDS) automation has the potential to improve the quality of the health care and patient safety. Essentially, CDS automation is a system that provides clinicians with computerized clinical data and is typically designed to aid decisionmaking in regards to clinical procedures. Unfortunately, CDS automation has not been fully implemented in ambulance care as it has yet to be integrated with the realities of clinical workflow. Methods already exist to measure the workflow and improving them, and these methods can be implemented in order to implement CDS automation and make sure that CDS automation works at the right time for the range of its users.

Kelly, K.M. "Building an Ambulance: ~~ambulance manufacturing is as much about design, engineering and technology as it is durability and functionality~~." Automotive Design & Production, April 2009, 121(4).

*ABSTRACT: Braun Industries in Van Wert, OH, manufactures up to 350 ambulances each year for some of the largest municipal fleets in the country, including Chicago, Boston and Miami-Dade. Since the needs of each fire department and non-municipal customer differ, the company's applications engineering department must pay careful attention identifying the equipment and layout needed to fulfill customer requirements--down to the location of oxygen outlets, auxiliary control panels and cabinetry--a process that requires working with more than 600 medical and safety equipment suppliers. Once the details have been nailed down, the design engineering group uses SolidWorks to develop 3D CAD files outlining the exact number of pieces needed--anywhere from 300 to more than 900-to build the box that is fitted on the back of the cab. Concurrently, electrical engineers verify the equipment selected by the customer will work within Braun's peer-to-peer multiplex electrical architecture. Once the design has been approved, the fabrication department converts the SolidWorks files onto SigmaNest, which automatically optimizes the layout of parts on each of the 2.4 m (8 ft) and 3.66 m (12 ft) sheets of 3.175 mm (1/8 in) thick marine-grade aluminum, reducing waste and improving efficiency. The parts are cut with a plasma torch, Trumpf punch or Komo router, then brake formed; it takes an average of 4 hours to cut as many as 80 sheets of parts for each box. The use of SigmaNest also allows Braun to store detailed specifications for each truck in a database for reference in case replacement parts need to be fabricated on short notice. All of the pieces are sent to the welding shop where they are spot welded together by hand, completing the basic box assembly. Then it moves onto paint. The box moves to final assembly, where lean manufacturing principles are followed. The 10219.3 sq meters (110000 sq ft) assembly hall is arranged by "value streams": chassis prep, fabrication and quality. The combined chassis and box--now called an "ambulance"-travel through the assembly process via a "work center" arrangement, defined as specific areas of assembly, such as electrical or upholstery. Parts are kitted by truck number and delivered line-side for each of the work centers; there are up to five work centers per assembly station. Once the kitted parts are placed on the truck, the ambulance is moved to the next station, where another work center is completed. The entire build process, from the first cut of aluminum to the final quality check, takes up to 35 days, with cost ranging from $85000 to $350000.

Levick, N.R. "Emergency Medical Services: A Unique Transportation Safety Challenge." Paper presented at the Transportation Research Board's 87th Annual Meeting, Washington DC, 2008.
*ABSTRACT: Emergency Medical Service (EMS) is an essential and transportation based emergency service, and now key component of the new SAFETEA-LU required State Strategic Highway Safety Plans. Ground EMS responds to approximately 30 million emergency medical/injury calls annually. In contrast to other commercial transport vehicles, ambulance transport safety is not currently encompassed by the Federal Motor Carrier Safety Administration (FMCSA), nor formally by any other overseeing body and hence the safety oversight of this transport system is fragmented and largely devoid of current

technical transportation safety input. This is of serious concern, particularly when the crash fatality rate for these EMS vehicles per mile traveled is estimated to be in excess of 10 fold higher than that for heavy trucks. Additionally there are ambulance 'wake effect' crashes, with rates in excess of five fold of the identified ambulance crash rates. These deficiencies in EMS transportation safety process range in spectrum from safety performance data capture, to transportation system safety engineering, and vehicle design, vehicle safety performance and occupant protection. There is also no process for formal knowledge transfer of existing transportation safety understanding and expertise or vehicle design and safety technical expertise either from the commercial vehicle industry or the automotive safety industry to the ambulance industry. This paper identifies some of the unique challenges of this EMS transportation system and addresses existing and innovative approaches for augmenting knowledge transfer potential from other transportation areas to enhance the safety of this special transportation system.

Nunnally, M., C.P. Nemeth, V. Brunetti, and R. Cook. "Lost in Menuspace: User Interactions with Complex Medical Devices." IEEE Transactions on Systems, Man and Cybernetics, Part A: Systems and Humans, 2004, 34(6): pp 736-742.
*ABSTRACT: The advent of fast-acting drugs has made the infusion pump the most pervasive electronic medical device in the acute care (hospital) environment. Despite the importance of its correct operation, incident reports in the US Food and Drug Administration (FDA) database implicate interface programming as a significant aspect of adverse outcomes. This article describes a study of infusion pump-programming performance by experienced healthcare professionals in a major urban teaching hospital. Early findings indicate that practitioner experience with device programming does not increase proficiency. This suggests that a complex menu structure ("menuspace") makes programming difficult and inefficient in ways that impede practitioner development of mental models that are sufficient for reliable device operation. This causes operators to become disoriented in the interface structure, or "lost in menuspace." We relate these findings to the current study of the USFDA adverse events reports and indicate directions for further research.

Paul, S.A., M. Reddy, and J. Abraham. "Collaborative Sensemaking during Emergency Crisis Response: How do ICTs help?" Poster presented at GROUP 2007, Sanibel Island, Florida, 2007.
*ABSTRACT: Sensemaking is the process of understanding an unfamiliar situation in order to act effectively. Crisis response requires emergency departments and emergency medical services teams to collaboratively make sense of an uncertain and unfamiliar situation. We conducted focus groups to examine how information and communication technologies help collaborative sensemaking across response teams. We found that communication of information was a key aspect of sensemaking and communication tools like the radio, phones, pagers, and paper were preferred to computer-based systems for

sensemaking among teams. Our findings highlight the need to develop new information systems, or enhance existing ones, for supporting collaborative sensemaking among geographically-distributed teams engaged in time-critical work.

Paxton, J.A. "Improving the Safety of EMS Personnel in the Patient Compartment of Violet Township Fire Department EMS Transport Vehicles." A research project submitted to the Ohio Fire Executive Fire Program, July 15, 2009.
*ABSTRACT: The problem this study will investigate is how to safely secure Violet Township Fire Department (VTFD) personnel during EMS transports, while maintaining sufficient operational mobility. The purpose of this project is to identify and to describe restraint options that will guide the VTFD in decision making that can improve the safety of crew members while performing patient care during EMS transport. The research design consisted of three segments: an internal survey of the VTFD membership, the review of the current styles and trends in ambulance manufacturing, and an examination of the ambulances of neighboring jurisdictions.

RESEARCH QUESTIONS: The following questions will be answered by this evaluative research: (1) What options are available to restrain EMS/firefighter personnel, while still allowing the needed mobility for patient care? (2) What are other fire departments doing to address this same problem? (3) What can the VTFD do to improve the safety of its current EMS transport vehicles? (4) What engineering options are available and could be utilized to provide increased occupant safety in future VTFD EMS transport vehicles?

The internal survey identified the occupational habits and tendencies of the VTFD EMS crews. The survey identified that the EMS crews in the VTFD ambulances were riding in the side-facing bench seats 93 % of the time. The survey further found mobility as the factor most likely to dictate seatbelt use by the patient attendant during transport. There was a 35 % reduction in seatbelt usage when transporting critical or unstable patients. The answers to the survey remained largely unaffected by time on the department or years of EMS experience. A review of several ambulance manufacturers found growing trends towards the development of safer vehicles. A look at nearby fire departments revealed few safety enhancements to their ambulances.

Recommendations for improving crewmember safety during EMS transport: (1) Upgrade the existing lap belt restraints in the current medics. (2) Continue researching ways to improve existing and future EMS vehicles. (3) Establish a committee to redesign the VTFD ambulance of the future. (4) Increase education/awareness of the VTFD. (5) Incorporate emergency vehicle driver's training into the department's routine. (6) Adjust the placement of supplies and equipment in the current ambulances to reflect the needs and or limitations of a single attendant.

Poulymenopoulou, M., F. Malamateniou, and G. Vassilacopoulos. "Specifying workflow process requirements for an emergency medical service." Journal of Medical Systems, 2003, 27(4): pp 325-335.

*ABSTRACT: Recent trends in healthcare delivery have led to a gradual shift in the conceptualization of healthcare information systems towards supporting healthcare processes in a more direct way. The move towards integrated and managed care, which requires designing healthcare processes around patient needs and incorporating efficiency considerations has led to an increased interest in process-oriented healthcare information systems based on workflow technology. This means to actively deliver the tasks to be performed to the right persons at the right time with the necessary information and the application functions needed. Moreover, workflow technology promotes a component-oriented development whereby the process logic is separated from application logic. This paper presents an approach to capturing process logic requirements for healthcare workflow systems with a view to design a system that is easily adjustable to process changes and to evolving organizational structures at a reasonable cost.

Snook, R., and R. Pacifico. "Ambulance ride: fixed or floating stretcher?" British Medical Journal, 1976, 2: pp 405-407.
*ABSTRACT: The alternatives of a purpose-built ambulance and a specially designed stretcher suspension system were considered and the features of the latter assessed by subjective and objective tests. The results showed a significant improvement in the quality of the ride offered to the patient.

3.6 Overall Design Evaluations and Examples

Bothwell, P.W. "An ambulance designed for the patient and crew." Public Health, 1960, 74(12): pp 459-464.
*ABSTRACT: An ambulance should be regarded as an important piece of specialized medical equipment and should be designed as such. It is of as much importance to get this piece of "socio-medical" apparatus correctly designed as it is to have correctly designed electrocardiographs, X-ray apparatus and electroencephalographs. All these pieces of equipment required combined medical and technical attention to suit them to their tasks. Ambulances exist for patients and crew, operate in society, and need to be designed accordingly.
A brief account is given of an ambulance design in which the above considerations have been kept in mind and the layout of the proposed suspension and lowering mechanism is shown diagrammatically. Reference is made to the general need to study the human engineering aspects of "socio-medical apparatus".

EMS World. "Next Generation Ambulance Puts Safety First." Accessed July 20, 2011. http://www.emsworld.com/print/EMS-World/Next-Generation-Ambulance-Puts-Safety-First/1$2481.
ABSTRACT: The American Medical Response (AMR) and the American Emergency Vehicles collaborated and presented a second-generation ambulance safety vehicle, called the Concept Ambulance-II or C2, in the 2005 EMS Expo. It boasts safety features such as two external cameras that allow the driver to monitor blind spots from the cab, and rear crew seats that are strategically located for optimal patient care and configured with four different types of safety harnesses that don't inhibit that care. All have five- or six-point harness systems that lock during sudden deceleration; cargo nets installed along internal voids, such as the curbside door well, to stop providers from striking the bulkhead; locking docking ports to secure patient-compartment equipment like EKG (electrocardiograph) monitor/defibrillators and eliminate "missiles" in a crash. Furthermore, it boasts all extra oxygen tanks being stored externally; turn-signal indicators and brake lighting installed in the back of the ambulance to warn providers delivering patient care of changes in direction and braking; a "black box" on-board computer system that records vehicle speed, monitors driving behavior and warns the driver about maneuvers that exceed preset safety parameters; reflective paint to make the vehicle more conspicuous; and a unique lighting package that includes amber caution lights that flash at motorists' eye level, LED emergency warning lights and under-body illumination. The price tag is about $200000, which is approximately 100 % higher than normal ambulance vehicles.

Hignett, S., E. Crumpton, and R. Coleman. "Designing emergency ambulances for the 21st century." Emergency Medicine Journal, 2009, 26(1): pp 135-140.
*ABSTRACT: BACKGROUND: In 2005 the Department of Health set out a vision

for the provision of future ambulance services with an increasing range of quality mobile healthcare services for patients with urgent and emergency care needs. This paper describes a scoping study funded by the National Patient Safety Agency and Ambulance Service Association to investigate the short and longer term requirements of future emergency ambulances. METHOD: Four stakeholder workshops were held to explore the wishes, concerns and preferences of the clinicians, operational staff and manufacturers about the future provision of ambulance services and problems and possible solutions relating to ambulance design and use. Incident reports relating to ambulance design and use were reviewed from three national and international databases. RESULTS: Nine design challenges were identified: access/egress; space and layout; securing people and equipment in transit; communication; security, violence and aggression; hygiene; equipment; vehicle engineering; patient experience. These were validated at the national UK ambulance conference (AMBEX 2006) with a rating questionnaire. CONCLUSION: The results are being used in the development of a national specification for future UK emergency ambulances.

Levick, N.R., and R. Grzebieta. "Ambulance vehicle crashworthiness and passive safety design -- A comparative evaluation of Australian and USA design and testing standards." Presentation given at the 12th International Conference on Emergency Medicine, San Francisco, California, April 3-4, 2008.
*ABSTRACT: Ambulances are largely exempt from crashworthiness and occupant protection passive safety design standards in the USA, and have a poor road safety record. This comparative evaluation of USA 'concept safety' ambulances and a standard Australian ambulance is based on basic principles of crashworthiness and available crash test data. There are features of USA ambulance design that are not within known principles and technical aspects of crashworthiness and safety design, and include some predictable serious occupant protection hazards. The USA ambulance industry should recognize and apply crashworthiness and occupant protection principles to reduce current system failures for this fleet of essential service vehicles.

Levick, N.R., and R. Grzebieta. "Crashworthiness Analysis of Three Prototype Ambulance Vehicles." Paper presented at the 20th International Technical Conference on the Enhanced Safety of Vehicles Conference (ESV: Enhanced Safety of Vehicles) in Lyon, France, June 18-21, 2007.
*ABSTRACT: This paper is an evaluation of the predicted safety performance of three USA prototype ambulance vehicles with aftermarket structural modifications. Expected safety performance was analyzed using existing and established automotive safety principles. Information on design and construction of the vehicles was identified, and evaluated via application of basic engineering crashworthiness principles and laws of physics, with a specific focus on countermeasure design for reducing harmful loading and injury causation potential in crashes or sudden decelerations. Data sources used for the analysis

included: vehicle specifications, inspections, photographs, crash tests and published crashworthiness and injury mitigation literature. Results demonstrated poor vehicle structural integrity and crashworthiness for these aftermarket modified ambulance vehicles. Assessed crashworthiness performance and occupant protection do not appear optimized even for the minimally structurally modified van. Current interior design features (seat design, patient transport device design, head strike zones and restraint systems) and layout, demonstrated predictable serious crashworthiness and occupant protection hazards. These are projected findings, rather than actual crashworthiness tests – however this is the first comparative automotive safety evaluation of prototype ambulance vehicles. This is key information for a major fleet of vehicles globally which has had minimal automotive safety attention or input to date. From this study it appears there are major deficiencies in safety design of these prototypes. Emphasis on a passenger compartment that has crashworthy features, effective seat design, based on existing literature and a clear focus on occupant human factors and equipment location and anchors, could provide for major safety enhancements for ambulance vehicles. There is need for vehicle safety researchers, ambulance industry and vehicle designers to recognize and apply these existing principles to reduce current failures in an important and essential service that appears to have a poor safety record, considerably below that of other passenger (Maguire 2003, Ray 2005, Levick 2006) and also other commercial vehicles (FMCSA).

Medtec Ambulance Corporation. ActionSafe Interior Configuration. Goshen, IN : Medtec Ambulance Corporation.
ABSTRACT: This is a redesign of the interior ambulance patient compartment layout that reduces the need of the Emergency Medical Service (EMS) worker's movements around in the compartment. According to Medtec, their ActionSafe interior configuration is designed to maximize the EMS working environment by: incorporating 5-point safety harnesses, keeping equipment and controls at arm's reach, increasing head space, adding padding throughout the compartment, and tapering and flaring cabinets away from impact zones.

National Patient Safety Agency (UK). Design for Patient Safety: Future Ambulances. NRLS 0463.
*ABSTRACT: The purpose of this joint National Patient Safety Agency (NPSA) and Helen Hamlyn Trust report is to promote discussion and innovative decision-making by NHS ambulance trusts in England and Wales, and to provide the NHS Purchasing and Supply Agency (PaSA) with safety criteria for the purchasing of ambulances. The NHS ambulance services are undergoing rapid change and modernisation, providing an opportunity for a servicewide approach to design and procurement to enhance safety.
The report sets out a three-stage design direction, for implementation over the next five to 10 years, to support standardisation and improvement of vehicle design; ensure equipment reliability and compatibility; and subsequently meet the evolving demands on NHS ambulance services.

National Patient Safety Agency (UK). Designing Future Ambulance Transport for Patient Safety: Research Undertaken. NRLS 0465.
*ABSTRACT: This first scoping study aims to investigate the developing models of service provision and the short and long term requirements of vehicles and equipment that will be needed to address the concerns of patient and staff safety in the future in the Ambulance Service. Three types of data were collected: archival incident reports, research literature and empirical data from workshops. The archival data were collected from three sources about reported incidents relating to ambulance, ambulance equipment design and use, and patient and staff safety. The research literature review was used to not only set out the background context but also to develop the conceptual framework for the analysis of the workshop data. Empirical data were collected from four user workshops. A dataset of 1352 incidents was received from the National Reporting and Learning System (NRLS) database and 1259 were retrieved from the Manufacturer and User facility Device Experience (MAUDE) database. Ten ambulance trusts responded to a request for information (from the 32 trusts contacted). After the analysis of the workshop data, the incident reports were reviewed and coded into the nine design challenges: Access/egress; space and layout; securing people and equipment in transit; communication; security, violence, and aggression; hygiene; equipment; vehicle engineering; patient experience. The data from the workbooks at the strategic workshop were analyzed thematically to identify six core areas of service provision. These areas of service provision were used as the discussion framework at the manufacturer and operational workshops. The data from the operational workshops were coded in two stages to allow for iterative analysis and further exploration of codes and themes. The coding by Roger Coleman/Merih Kunur resulted in two distinct design outputs for (1) design issues and (2) problems/ features. These codes were then scrutinized by Emma Crumpton, resulting in the 31 codes. At this stage a detailed secondary coding was conducted within the codes to identify nine higher level codes and address duplication between codes (Emma Crumpton/Sally Halls). These design challenges were further checked against the primary coding by Sally Halls to confirm inclusiveness. There was found to be a divergence between the NRLS data and the incidents reported by the individual trusts for some of the design challenges, for example securing people and equipment in transit, and equipment. There are a number of possible causes for this divergence, including the design of the NRLS interface and subsequent data input. Particular areas needing further research are communication, hygiene and the patient experience.

Van Gogh, D., K. Kawakami, and H. Shimizu. "Design Concept of Electric Vehicle Ambulance." Journal of Asian Electric Vehicles, 2005, 3(1): pp 713-719.
*ABSTRACT: Today's emergency transportation by internal combustion engine ambulances has many problems: it has a high vibration for the patient and the medics, it has a limited size of workstation for the medical treatment, it slowly

accelerates with jolts and it has a high floor base which makes driving unstable while cornering. An Electric Vehicle ambulance, EV ambulance, is proposed to solve all this problems. The structural design of today's ambulance is compared with the design concept of an EV ambulance. The EV component technologies of an in-wheel drive, component built-in frame and tandem suspension system are applied to the EV ambulance. Four types of ambulances are presented: one based upon the average outer dimensions of a conventional ambulance, second based upon the average inner dimensions of workspace of the medics, third with a driver seat in the middle of the cabin and finally with a driver seat on an elevated position. A dual direction drive is applied in the ambulance and one type of EV ambulance its length is reduced to 2 m so that it can enter into buildings. The EV ambulances illustrate that a smooth vibration and high acceleration of 0.4 g-force (gravitational force) is reached, the noise inside the cabin is reduced from 90 dbA to 60 dbA; the floor height is reduced from 50 cm to 30 cm, 85 % of the total inner space can be used as a workspace, and stable drive and cornering is most efficient during an emergency transportation.

3.7 Securing People & Equipment

Becker, L.R., E. Zaloshnja, N.R. Levick, G. Li, and T.R. Miller. "Relative risk of injury and death in ambulances and other emergency vehicles." Accidenty Analysis & Prevention, November 2003, 35(6): pp 941-948.
*ABSTRACT: This study addresses of the impacts of emergency vehicle (ambulances, police cars and fire trucks) occupant seating position, restraint use and vehicle response status on injuries and fatalities. Multi-way frequency and ordinal logistic regression analyses were performed on two large national databases, the National Highway Traffic Safety Administration's Fatality Analysis Reporting System (FARS) and the General Estimates System (GES). One model estimated the relative risk ratios for different levels of injury severity to occupants traveling in ambulances. Restrained ambulance occupants involved in a crash were significantly less likely to be killed or seriously injured than unrestrained occupants. Ambulance rear occupants were significantly more likely to be killed than front-seat occupants. Ambulance occupants traveling non-emergency were more likely than occupants traveling emergency to be killed or severely injured. Unrestrained ambulance occupants, occupants riding in the patient compartment and especially unrestrained occupants riding in the patient compartment were at substantially increased risk of injury and death when involved in a crash. A second model incorporated police cars and fire trucks. In the combined ambulance-fire truck-police car model, the likelihood of an occupant fatality for those involved in a crash was higher for routine responses. Relative to police cars and fire trucks, ambulances experienced the highest percentage of fatal crashes where occupants are killed and the highest percentage of crashes where occupants are injured. Lack of restraint use and/or responding with 'lights and siren' characterized the vast majority of fatalities among fire truck occupants. A third model incorporated non-special use van and passenger car occupants, which otherwise replicated the second model. Our findings suggest that ambulance crewmembers riding in the back and firefighters in any seating position, should be restrained whenever feasible. Family members accompanying ambulance patients should ride in the front-seat of the ambulance.

Green, J.D., D.E. Ammons, A.J. Isaacs, P.H. Moore, R.L. Whisler, and J.E. White. "Creating a Safe Work Environment for Emergency Medical Service Workers." Paper presented for Proceedings ASSE Professional Development Conference and Exposition, June 9-12, 2008.
*ABSTRACT: Seat belts are required in U.S. ambulances, as with other motor vehicles manufactured in accordance with the current Federal Motor Vehicle Safety Standards (FMVSS), as regulated by the National Highway Traffic Safety Administration (NHTSA). These regulations are also cited in the Specification for the Star of Life Ambulance, KKK-A-1822F, as issued by the General Services Administration (GSA), which is widely adopted as the defacto industry specification for ambulances. The required occupant restraints do not allow emergency medical service (EMS) workers the mobility required to care for

patients. As a result, EMS workers routinely work unrestrained in the patient compartment, daily risking their safety and health in the care of others. In an effort to solve this problem for existing and new ambulances alike, NIOSH (National Institute of Occupational Safety and Health) tested four different retrofittable restraint systems, each which improved crash protection for the worker while allowing mobility needed to provide patient care. In parallel, the City of Winter Park (Florida) Fire and Rescue Department (WPFD), in collaboration with Medtec Ambulance Corporation, has designed and fielded a new ambulance patient compartment that significantly reduces the need for the EMS worker to move from a seated position to care for the patient. Together, these two work environment changes represent unique opportunities to substantially improve worker safety without compromising patient care. The objective of this research study was to utilize digital human modeling tools to evaluate reach envelopes for three different human body sizes (5th percentile female, as well as, the 50th and 95th percentile male: by stature and weight), when positioned in two different commercially available ambulance patient compartments. The evaluation was expanded to test each body size, in each environment, using two different restraint systems: one fixed and one allowing mobility, if needed, to assess the ability of a worker to care for the patient and reach equipment while remaining restrained. The underlying premise is that it is better to be restrained than unrestrained, and further, it is better to be restrained and seated than restrained and out of the seat. Results from this study illustrate the strengths and limitations of the patient compartment configuration in an ambulance built and fielded in accordance with the current FMVSS and the Federal Specification for the Star of Life Ambulance, KKK-A-1822E, as issued by the General Services Administration (GSA). This study also discusses potential improvements to the safety and health of EMS workers, if NIOSH tested mobile restraint systems, which increase reach envelope while allowing EMS workers to remain restrained, were adopted. The approach taken by the WPFD to redesign the work environment by substantially reducing the need for mobility, thus allowing EMS workers to remain seated and restrained for the majority of their work tasks, offers a real opportunity to improve the safety of ambulances to be fielded in the future if this design were to be adopted. Finally, the WPFD (Winter park Fire Department) design when coupled with a mobile restraint offers the best of both designs.

Green, J.D., J.R. Yannaccone, R.S. Current, L.A. Sicher, P.H. Moore, and G.R. Whitman. "Assessing the performance of various restraints on ambulance patient compartment workers during crash events."
International Journal of Crashworthiness, 2010, 15(5): pp 517-541.
*ABSTRACT: The inability of emergency medical service (EMS) workers to remain safely restrained while treating patients in the patient compartment of a moving ambulance has been identified as a key impediment to EMS worker safety in North America. It has been hypothesized that restraint systems designed to provide mobility while offering the ability to lock during an impact or sudden maneuver, could greatly enhance worker safety in the back of

ambulances. Through a series of 33 sled and crash tests impacting the front, side, and rear of simulated and actual ambulance patient compartments, the National Institute for Occupational Safety and Health examined the biomechanical and kinematic effects of two-, four- and five-point restraints on 95th percentile male Hybrid III anthropomorphic test devices. Results indicate that the inclusion of restraint systems offering mobility have the potential to improve worker safety under many working conditions in this unique work environment.

Green, J.D., P. Moore, R. Current, J. Yannaccone, G. Whitman, D. Day, S. Prooudfoot, T. Bobick, and N. Romano. "Reducing Vehicle Crash-Related EMS Worker Injuries through Improvements in Restraint Systems." Presented at the conference proceedings for the XVIIth World Safety Congress, Orlando, Florida, September 20, 2005.

ABSTRACT: The National Institute for Occupational Safety and Health (NIOSH), Division of Safety Research, collaborated with the U.S, Army Tank-Automotive and Armaments Command, the Canadian Forces Health Services Group Headquarters, the Ministry of Health & Long-Term Care, Ontario, Canada, and the U.S. Fire Administration on a research effort to increase the crash protection afforded emergency medical service (EMS) workers in ambulance patient compartments. The estimated fatality rate for EMS workers is 12.7 deaths per 100000 workers, more than twice the national average of 5.0 for all U.S. workers. Transportation-related events, including ambulance crashes, are the most common cause of death among U.S. EMS workers. Ambulance crash investigations from the National Highway Traffic Safety Administration (NHTSA) and NIOSH were used to identify injury risk and circumstances. Results of these investigations show that regardless of occupant location, non-use of occupant restraints resulting in collisions between unrestrained occupants and compartment bulkheads and cabinets is the primary injury risk.

Seat belts currently provided in ambulances do not allow the mobility that EMS workers need to care for patients. As a result, EMS workers routinely work unrestrained in the patient compartment. Occupant restraints that provide mobility within the ambulance patient compartment, and are capable of mitigating crash-related injuries were evaluated using a mathematical model; a 29-run, laboratory-based, sled-testing program; and, a four-vehicle crash-test program. Each sled and crash test included four instrumented anthropomorphic test devices (ATDs) or crash test dummies. During these tests, the mobile restraints prevented the ATDs from secondary collisions in the patient compartment and were structurally sound at acceleration levels between 25 g-forces and 30 f-forces. Use of mobile restraints has the potential to significantly reduce crash-related injuries to EMS workers in ambulance patient compartments.

Recognizing seat belts have been viewed as an impediment to the ability of EMS workers to provide patient care, future NIOSH work with mobile restraints will focus on factors that affect user acceptance.

Larmon, B., T.L. LeGassick, and D.L. Schringer. "Differential front and back seat safety belt use by prehospital care providers." The American Journal of Emergency Medicine, 1993, 11: pp 595-599.
*ABSTRACT: The object of the study was to assess the habits and attitudes of prehospital care personnel regarding safety belt use in the front and rear ambulance compartments. Therefore, a cross-sectional descriptive survey was administered at emergency medical service conferences and through provider agencies throughout the United States and Canada. Approximately 900 public, private, and volunteer prehospital care providers participated. Demographic information, traffic collision history, percent of time safety belts were used, belief in safety belt use, and reasons for nonuse in the rear compartment of the ambulance were measured. The results showed that safety belt use was highest in the front seat during emergency runs (median, 100 %) and rarest in the back compartment during emergency runs (median, 0 %). Respondents cited the following reasons for non-use in the rear compartment: inhibited patient care (67.9 %), restricted movement (34.7 %) inconvenience (15.1 %), or lack of efficacy (5.3 %). Prehospital care personnel typically wear safety belts when in the front seat, but not while in the rear compartment of the ambulance. More intensive efforts at educating prehospital care providers about the importance of safety restraints in the rear compartment, enumerating patient care activities that can be performed while wearing a safety belt, and design of a functional restraint system for the rear compartment may increase ambulance safety.

Levick, N.R., G. Li, and J. Yannaccone. "Biomechanics of the Patient Compartment of Ambulance Vehicles under Crash Conditions: Testing Countermeasures to Mitigate Injury." Paper presented at the SAE 2001 World Congress, Detroit, Michigan, March 2001. doi: 10.4271/2001-01-1173.
*ABSTRACT: There has been very limited research on the biomechanics of occupant safety in the ambulance environment. Occupant protection or crash testing safety standards for these unique vehicles are lacking in the United States. Recent studies have identified ambulances as high risk passenger transport vehicles. This study was conducted to identify some of the occupant safety hazards in the ambulance environment and to determine the efficacy of some countermeasures to mitigate ambulance occupant injury. Accelerator sled testing of the ambulance rear patient compartment (ambulance box or rear cabin) with Anthropomorphic Test Devices was conducted under frontal impact conditions with a target sled pulse was 26 g-forces and 48.28 kp/h (30 mph). The ambulance box was configured with instrumented and uninstrumented Anthropomorphic Test Devices positioned as in the real world environment. Two uninstrumented 95% Hybrid-II Anthropomorphic Test Devices were lap belted and positioned in the occupant compartment, one on the rear-facing attendant's seat and one on the side-facing bench seat. A Side Impact Dummy was unbelted, seated on the front of the side-facing bench seat and positioned next to a passive restraint device. An instrumented Hybrid-III 3 year old child Anthropomorphic Test Device was restrained in a child restraint system, secured to the gurney via a dual belt path. The actual sled pulse achieved was 34 g-

forces and 55.26 kp/h (34.34 mph), and due to separation of the ambulance box from the chassis/sled, the crash pulse imparted to the patient compartment were 20 g-forces and 33.64 kp/h (20.9 mph). Head Injury Criterion (HIC) values calculated for the restrained Hybrid-III child Anthropomorphic Test Device were 171, however for the unbelted Side Impact Dummy the HIC was projected to be in excess of 1000. Although this study was a preliminary study, the findings confirmed that there are unique occupant hazards in the ambulance vehicle environment and that certain restraint practices are of value and that some injury mitigating countermeasures are ineffective. Importantly this study also demonstrated the potential for unrestrained occupants to be not only a hazard to themselves but also a hazard to the restrained occupants in the ambulance patient compartment. This study highlights the need for the development of dynamic safety standards for occupant restraint in this environment.

Levick, N.R., and M.A. Garigan. "Solution to Head Injury Protection for Emergency Medical Service Providers." Paper presented at the proceedings for the International Ergonomics Association, Maastricht, the Netherlands, July 2006.
*ABSTRACT: The purpose of this study is to identify applicable standards and potential devices for head protection for the ground ambulance transport environment. Occupational health and safety standards for Head Protection for Emergency Medical Service (EMS) providers in USA, Australia and Europe were reviewed. Existing helmets intended for, or adopted for use by EMS personnel were identified, and unique design elements determined via focus groups and expert panels. The findings demonstrated that there are no USA head protection standards for this population, although such standards exist in Australia and Europe. Unique design features, suggested by providers were: communications capability (with patients, 85 %; and driver 69 %) and stethoscope auscultation (89 %); Expert panels added: Effective in high horizontal g-forces; Identify the responder; Biohazard protection and Image enhancing. Although there is demonstrated risk for serious and/or fatal head impacts in the ambulance environment, there is an absence of standards or guidelines for occupational head protection, for USA ground EMS providers. An head protection device should include communication capacity, and address comfort, visibility and aesthetics and be protective for automotive crash forces.

Rolandelli, P.J. "Adjustable safety seat for ambulances and other emergency vehicles." US Patent 4251100 filed May 11, 1979 and issued February 17, 1981.
*ABSTRACT: An adjustable safety seat is provided to enhance the ability of medical attendants to perform emergency medical services on a patient in a moving ambulance or other emergency vehicle. An adjustable seat, backrest and restraint for use with center-mounted cots in an emergency vehicle enable one medical attendant to perform, without interruption, the chest compressions and ventilations required for cardiopulmonary resuscitation, while simultaneously

protecting the attendant from falls and possible injury when the vehicle is in motion. The adjustable safety seat enables the attendant to assume the optimal position for performing cardiopulmonary resuscitation. When not required for cardiopulmonary resuscitation, the seat can be adjusted to facilitate performance of other medical services on the patient.

Stanley, L., and R. Kline. "Naturalistic safety evaluation of a medic's work environment during rural emergency response." Presentation given at the Transportation Research Board Annual Meeting, January, 2011.
ABSTRACT: In this presentation, the objectives and preliminary results for the project to increase medic and public safety through the collection and analysis of data. The primary objectives of the project is to determine the rate of restraint use by emergency medical service (EMS) workers, determine significant causes leading to medics being unrestrained, identify medic activities and physical hardships imposed by their equipments or procedures, determine biomechanical forces experienced by medics during patient transport, and identify factors that influence ambulance travel in emergency mode. After describing the methods of collecting and analyzing data, the presentation shows some results for restraint usage (average of 2.6 % of the time restrained per trip), reach analysis (20 unique reaches identified), and the fact that the vibrant exposure is at normal standard (based on the International Organization of Standardization Standard, ISO STD 2361) levels.

Studnek, J.R., and A. Ferketich. "Organizational policy and other factors associated with emergency medical technician seat belt use." Journal of Safety Research, 2007, 38: pp 1-8.
*ABSTRACT: INTRODUCTION: The purpose of this study was to determine factors associated with seat belt usage among Emergency Medical Technicians (EMTs). METHODS: As part of biennial re-registration paperwork, nationally registered EMTs completed a survey on the safety and health risks facing Emergency Medical Services (EMS) providers. Respondents were asked to describe their seat belt use while in the front seats of an ambulance. They were categorized as "high" in seat belt use if it had been more than a year since they had not worn their seat belt or "low" in seat belt use if they had not worn their seat belt at least once within the past 12 months. A logistic regression model was fit to estimate the association between seat belt use, organizational seat belt policy, type of EMS organization worked for, EMT certification level, and the size of community where EMS work is performed. RESULTS: Of the 41,823 EMTs that re-registered in 2003, surveys were received from 29,575 (70.7 %). A significant interaction between organizational seat belt policy and type of EMS organization was found to exist. Participants reporting no organizational seat belt policy had lower odds of seat belt usage when compared to individuals that do have a seat belt policy. Odds Ratios ranged from 0.20 (95 % CI 0.1-0.4) for military organization to 0.59 (95 % CI 0.38-0.93) for private EMS organizations. Paramedics and those working in rural areas also had lower odds of seat belt use. CONCLUSION: Several factors were found to be associated with seat belt

usage among EMTs while in the front compartment of an ambulance. However, it appears that only one, organizational policy, is a modifiable characteristic.

3.8 Standards & Guidelines

Ambulance Manufacturers Division. AMD Standards. 2007.
ABSTRACT: This United States standard establishes minimum requirements for performance tests for the safety of new ambulance motor vehicles and associated motor vehicle equipment. This standard works in conjunction with the Federal Specification for the Star-of-Life Ambulances, KKK-A-1822, in order to meet the performance testing requirements set in the Specification.

Ambulance Manufacturers Division. Proposed AMD Standard-Final Draft: Equipment Mounts and Cabinet Closures. 0027, 2011.
*ABSTRACT: SCOPE AND PURPOSE: This proposed document establishes a method for testing interior mounted equipment, cot-mounted equipment, and interior cabinet doors in ambulances. This is a type test. Cots/litters/gurneys are not included in this document. APPLICABILITY: This document applies to all interior/cot-mounting solutions for equipment in excess of 1.36 kilograms (three pounds), and to all interior cabinets and doors.

Ambulance Manufacturers Division. Proposed AMD Standard-Revision 11: Seat, Seat Mount and Occupant Restraint Dynamic Testing. 0026, 2010.
*ABSTRACT: SCOPE AND PURPOSE: This standard establishes minimum requirements for testing of all patient compartments designated seating positions, seat mounting systems, associated occupant restraints and belt mounting systems, either fabricated by an ambulance builder or acquired from a seat or restraint manufacturer. This is a type test. APPLICABILITY: This proposed standard applies to all patient compartment designated seating positions, seat mounting systems, and associated occupant restraints, whether part of the ambulance construction or manufactured by a third party for installation in ambulances.

Ambulance Manufacturers Division. Proposed Revision of AMD Standard: Method for Conducting Litter and Litter Retention System Dynamic Test. 004, 2010.
*ABSTRACT: SCOPE AND PURPOSE:This document establishes the method for testing the litter, litter retention system, and litter-based patient restraints when installed per the litter manufacturer's directions. This is a type test. APPLICABILITY: This proposed document applies to all litters, litter attaching hardware, and litter-based patient restraints manufactured for installation in ambulances.

ASTM International. Standard Guide for Training Emergency Medical Services Ambulance Operations. F1705-96, 2007.
*ABSTRACT: SCOPE: This guide provides minimum training standards for Emergency Medical Services (EMS) Ambulance Operators including legal aspects, operator qualifications and testing, history of EMS vehicle operations, vehicle types/equipment, safety, physical forces, mechanics, pre-run, operations, post-run, and special circumstances. This training guide promotes the safe and

efficient delivery of the ambulance, equipment, crew, passengers and patients, during all phases of the delivery of EMS involving the ambulance; at all times exercising the highest degree of care for the safety of the public. This standard may be applied to the driving of other EMS vehicles that do not necessarily provide patient transportation. This guide shall be used as the basis for all programs relevant to the training of the emergency medical services operators. This standard does not purport to address all of the safety concerns, if any, associated with its use. It is the responsibility of the user of this standard to establish appropriate safety and health practices and determine the applicability of regulatory limitations prior to use.

ASTM International. Standard Practice for Human Engineering Design for Marine Systems, Equipment, and Facilities. F1166-07, 2007.
*ABSTRACT: SCOPE: This practice provides ergonomic design criteria from a human-machine perspective for the design and construction of martime vessels and structures and for equipments, systems, and subsystems contained therein, including vendor-purchased hardware and software. The focus of these design criteria is on the design and evaluation of human-machine interfaces, including the interfaces between humans on the one side and controls and displays, physical environments, structures, consoles, panels and workstations, layout and arrangement of ship spaces, maintenance workplaces, labels and signage, alarms, computer screens, material handling, valves, and other specific equipments on the other. The criteria contained within this practice shall be applied to the design and construction of all hardware and software within a ship or maritime structure that the human crew members come in contact in any manner for operation, habitability, and maintenance purposes. Unless otherwise stated in specific provisions of a ship or maritime structure design contract or specification, this practice is to be used to design maritime vessels, structures, equipment, systems, and subsystems to fit the full potential user population range of 5 th % females to 95 th % males.

British Standards Institution. Medical Vehicles and Their Equipment - Road Ambulances. BS EN 1789:2007, 2007.
*ABSTRACT: SCOPE: This European Standard specifies requirements for the design, testing, performance and equipping of road ambulances used for the transport and care of patients. It contains requirements for the patient's compartment. This European Standard does not cover the requirements for approval and registration of the vehicle and the training of the staff which is the responsibility of the authority/authorities in the country where the ambulance is to be registered. This European Standard is applicable to road ambulances capable of transporting at least one person on a stretcher. Requirements are specified for categories of road ambulances based in increasing order of the level of treatment that can be carried out. These are the patient transport ambulance (types A1 A2), the emergency ambulance (type B) and the mobile intensive care unit (type C). This European Standard gives general requirements for Medical devices carried

in road ambulances and used therein and outside hospitals and clinics in situations where the ambient conditions can differ from normal indoor conditions.

Ministry of Health and Long-Term Care (Ontario, Canada). Ontario Provincial Land Ambulance & Emergency Response Vehicle Standard. Version 4.0, March 21, 2008.
*ABSTRACT: SCOPE OF THE STANDARD: This Standard describes the minimum acceptable requirements for land ambulances for use by an operator of a land ambulance service. Annex A of this standard describes the minimum acceptable requirements for emergency response vehicles intended for use in ambulance services in the Province of Ontario. Annex B of this standard describes the minimum acceptable requirements for the transfer of a Patient Compartment Module to another chassis intended for use in ambulance services in the Province of Ontario. Annex C of the standard is the Compliance Checklist for a new ambulance. Annex D of this standard is the Compliance Checklist for a remounted ambulance. Every operator of a land ambulance service shall be responsible for fully complying, or ensuring full compliance, with every provision of this Standard.

National Academy of Sciences - National Research Council, Washington, DC Division of Medical Sciences. Medical Requirements for Ambulance Design and Equipment. Emergency Health Series. PHS-Pub-1071-C-3, 1970.
*ABSTRACT: A vehicle must meet certain specific requirements to be classified as an ambulance if it is to satisfy the demands of the physician in terms of emergence care for which properly trained ambulance attendants can be held responsible. Developed by professional and lay experts for use by automotive designers and manufacturing, this publication would be useful resource material for a teacher in a technical institute or instructors of emergency squad personnel. Requirements are provided for: (1) The Ambulance, including requirements for general vehicular design and specific requirements for the driver and patient areas, (2) Security and Rescue Equipment, (3) Emergency Care Equipment and Supplies, which include litters, airway care, ventilation, oxygenation, external cardiac compression, immobilization of fractures, prevention and treatment of shock, wound dressings, emergency childbirth and transportation of newborn infants, poisoning, and special equipment, (4) Communication and Documentation, which includes a 2-way radio, telemetry equipment, and recording devices and (5) Transportation by Air.

National Fire Protection Association. Proposed Draft of NFPA 1917 Standard of Automotive Ambulances. NFPA1917, 2013.
*ABSTRACT: SCOPE: This standard establishes the minimum requirements for new automotive emergency medical services (EMS) ground vehicles used for out-of-hospital medical care and patient transport. Ther term 'new' as applied in this standard is intended to refer to the original construction of an ambulance using all new materials and parts. PUPOSE: The purpose of this document is to specify minimum requirements, performance parameters, and essential criteria

for the design of ground ambulances. APPLICATION: This standard shall apply equally to vehicles intended for use in both emergency and non-emergency operations. This standard shall not apply to the following: (1) Refurbished and re-mounted vehicles; (2) Vehicles that are used for transport of more than two stretcher-bound patients at the same time; (3) Mass casualty vehicles; (4) Military field ambulances; (5) Vehicles intended for use as fire apparatus as specified in NFPA 1901 and NFPA 1906.

National Highway Traffic Safety Administration, Washington, D.C. Ambulance Design Criteria. 1973.
*ABSTRACT: Indexed design and performance criteria for ambulances, developed by the National Academy of Engineering at the request of the National Highway Traffic Safety Administration, are presented. Part I of the report provides historical and technical background, and describes the need for standardization of ambulance design and performance. The purpose and scope of the study are discussed in terms of vehicles, vehicle elements, and vehicle characteristics. From the specific criteria detailed in Part II of the report, several recommendations selected for their special significance, are highlighted. These relate to the design of the patient compartment; standardization of ambulance manufacture; principal environmental requirements for medical care; communications requirements; national standardization of external identification; omission of windows in the patient compartment to enhance privacy and efficiency; adequate acceleration capability; and application of Federal Motor Vehicle Safety Standards appropriate for the kind of chassis employed. Vehicle characteristics for which standards could not be recommended due to lack of adequate objective data include: color and intensity of identification lights; riding quality and stability; noise and vibration; and vehicle braking system. A bibliography and a brief description of applicable Federal Motor Vehicle Safety Standards are appended.

Society of Automotive Engineers International. Surface Vehicle Recommended Practice: Occupant Restraint and Equipment Mounting Integrity – Frontal Impact System-Level Ambulance Patient Compartment. SAE J2917, 2010.
*ABSTRACT: SCOPE: This SAE Recommended Practice describes the test procedures for conducting frontal impact occupant restraint and equipment mounting integrity tests for ambulance patient compartment applications. Its purpose is to describe crash pulse characteristics and establish recommended test procedures that will standardize restraint system and equipment mounting testing for ambulances. Descriptions of the test set-up, test instrumentation, photographic/video coverage, and the test fixtures are included.

Society of Automotive Engineers International. Surface Vehicle Recommended Practice: Occupant Restraint and Equipment Mounting Integrity -- Side Impact System-Level Ambulance Patient Compartment. SAE J2956, 2010.

*ABSTRACT: This SAE Recommended Practice describes the test procedures for conducting side impact occupant restraint and equipment mounting integrity tests for ambulance patient compartment applications. Its purpose is to describe crash pulse characteristics and establish recommended test procedures that will standardize restraint system and equipment mounting testing for ambulances. Descriptions of the test set-up, test instrumentation, photographic/video coverage, and the test fixtures are included.

Standards Australia and Standards New Zealand. Australian/New Zealand Standards: Ambulance Restraint Systems. AS/NZS 4535, 1999.
*ABSTRACT: SCOPE: This Standard applies to motor vehicles designed as, or modified and converted into, ambulances for the transportation of occupants and equipment. The Standard specifies the requirements for restraining equipment and occupants sharing the same interior space. It may not be possible under all conditions to restrain occupants in the ideal configuration. OBJECTIVE: The objective of this Standard is to decrease the impact hazard to occupants during an accident whilst being transported in an ambulance.

U.S. General Services Administration. Federal Specification for the Star-of-Life Ambulance. KKK-A-1822F, 2007.
*ABSTRACT: PURPOSE: The purpose of this document is to describe ambulances that are authorized to display the "Star of Life" symbol. It establishes minimum specifications, performance parameters and essential criteria for the design of ambulances and to provide a practical degree of standardization. The object is to provide ambulances that are nationally recognized, properly constructed, easily maintained, and, when professionally staffed and provisioned, will function reliably in pre-hospital or other mobile emergency medical service.

4. ACRONYMS

AMBEX	National United Kingdom Ambulance Conference
AMD	Ambulance Manufacturers Division
AMR	American Medical Response
ASA	Ambulance Service Association (United Kingdom)
ATD	Anthropomorphic Test Dummy
CDC	Center for Disease Control
CDS	Clinical Decision Support
CEN	European Committee on Standardization
CPR	Cardiopulmonary Resuscitation
DOJ	United States Department of Justice
EKG	Electrocardiograph
EMS	Emergency Medical Services
EMT	Emergency Medical Technician
ESV	Enhanced Safety of Vehicles
FARS	Fatality Analysis Reporting System
FMCSA	Federal Motor Carrier Safety Administration
FMVSS	Federal Motor Vehicle Safety Standards
GES	General Estimates System
GSA	General Services Administration
ICU	Intensive Care Unit
IFSTA	International Fire Service Training Association
ISO STD	International Organization of Standardization
JEMS	JEMS: Journal of Emergency Medical Services
MIP	MIP: Mixed Integer Programming
NEISS	National Electronic Injury Surveillance System
NFPA	National Fire Protection Association
NHS	National Health Service
NHTSA	National Highway Traffic Safety Administration
NIJ	National Institute of Justice
NIOSH	National Institute of Occupational Safety and Health
NPSA	National Patient Safety Agency (United Kingdom)
NREMT	National Registry of Emergency Medical Technicians
NRLS	National Reporting and Learning Service (United Kingdom)
PaSA	Purchasing and Supply Agency (United Kingdom)
SAE	Society of Automotive Engineers
SAFETEA-LU	Safe, Accountable, Flexible, Efficient Transportation Equity Act: A Legacy for Users
STD	Standard
SUMMA 112	Medical Emergency Services of the Madrid, Spain Regional Government

USFA	United States Fire Administration
WPFD	Winter Park Fire Department
VTFD	Violet Township Fire Department

Acknowledgements

The US Department of Homeland Security Science and Technology Directorate (DHS S&T) Human Factors/Behavioral Sciences Division sponsored the production of this material under Interagency Agreement HSHQDC-11-X-00049 with the National Institute of Standards and Technology (NIST). The work described was funded by the United States Government and is not subject to copyright.

The authors of this report would like to thank Jennifer Marshall of NIST Office of Law Enforcement (OLES) and Jennifer Moore, Carlotta Boone, Allison Jacobs and Thomas Aten from BMT Designers & Planners for their help in compiling this report.

Disclaimer

Certain commercial equipment, instruments, or materials are identified in this paper to facilitate understanding. Such identification does not imply recommendation or endorsement by the National Institute of Standards and Technology, nor does it imply that the materials or equipment identified are necessarily the best available for the purpose.

www.ingramcontent.com/pod-product-compliance
Lightning Source LLC
Chambersburg PA
CBHW081738170526
45167CB00009B/3869